LOVE YOUR BODY
FEED YOUR SOUL

SELF-CARE RITUALS AND RECIPES FOR YOUR **INNER GODDESS**

SUMMER SANDERS

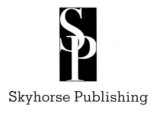

Skyhorse Publishing

Skyhorse Publishing books may be purchased in bulk at special discounts for sales promotion, corporate gifts, fund-raising, or educational purposes. Special editions can also be created to specifications. For details, contact the Special Sales Department, Skyhorse Publishing, 307 West 36th Street, 11th Floor, New York, NY 10018 or info@skyhorsepublishing.com.

Skyhorse® and Skyhorse Publishing® are registered trademarks of Skyhorse Publishing, Inc.®, a Delaware corporation.

Visit our website at www.skyhorsepublishing.com.

10 9 8 7 6 5 4 3 2 1

Library of Congress Cataloging-in-Publication Data is available on file.

Cover design by Daniel Brount
Cover photo by Lauren Schumacher

Print ISBN: 978-1-5107-4791-3
Ebook ISBN: 978-1-5107-4793-7

Printed in China

Neither the author or the publisher is engaged in rendering professional advice or services to the individual reader. The ideas, protocols, procedures, and suggestions in this book are not intended as a substitute for consulting with your physician. All matters regarding your health require medical supervision. Neither the author nor the publisher shall be liable or responsible for any loss or damage allegedly arising from any information or suggestion in the book.

The author or publisher is not responsible for your specific health or allergy needs that may require medical supervision. The publisher or author is not responsible for any adverse reactions to the recipes contained in this book.

Dedicated to you, dear reader, you are the inspiration and light of this world. I hope this book is a key to unlocking what already flows within, a river of depth, beauty, and health.

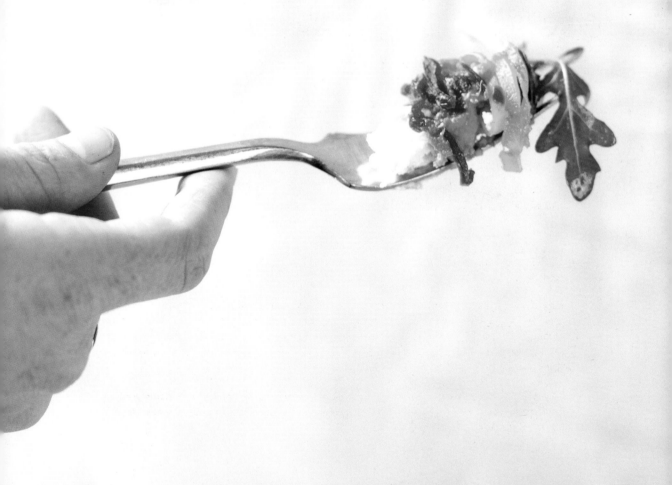

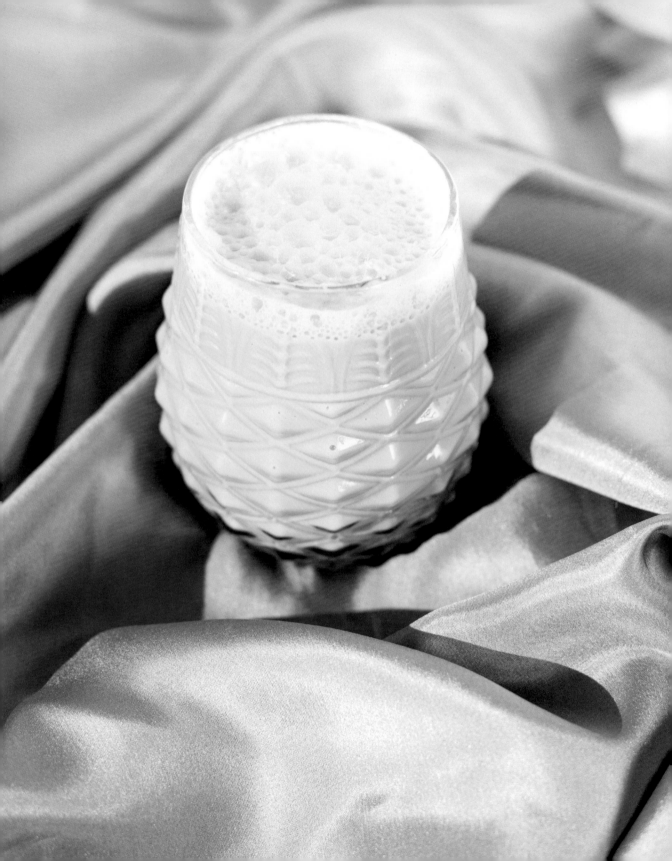

CONTENTS

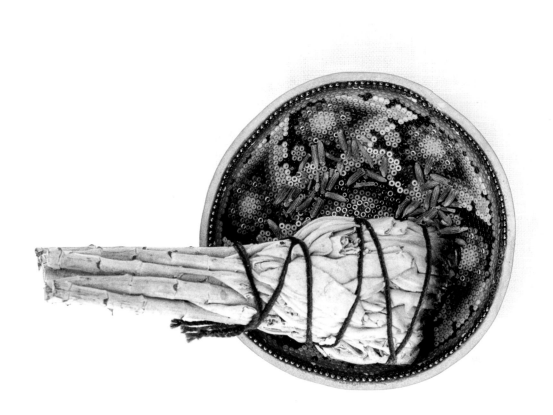

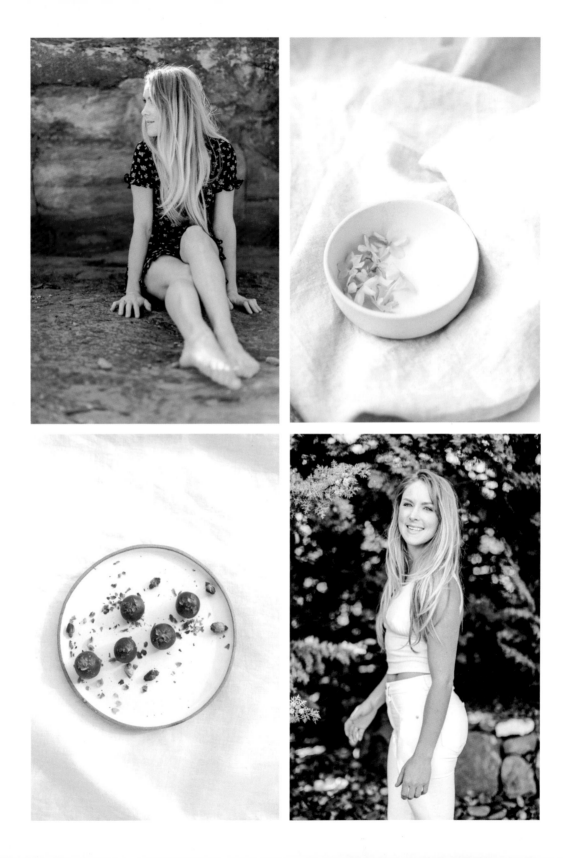

INTRODUCTION

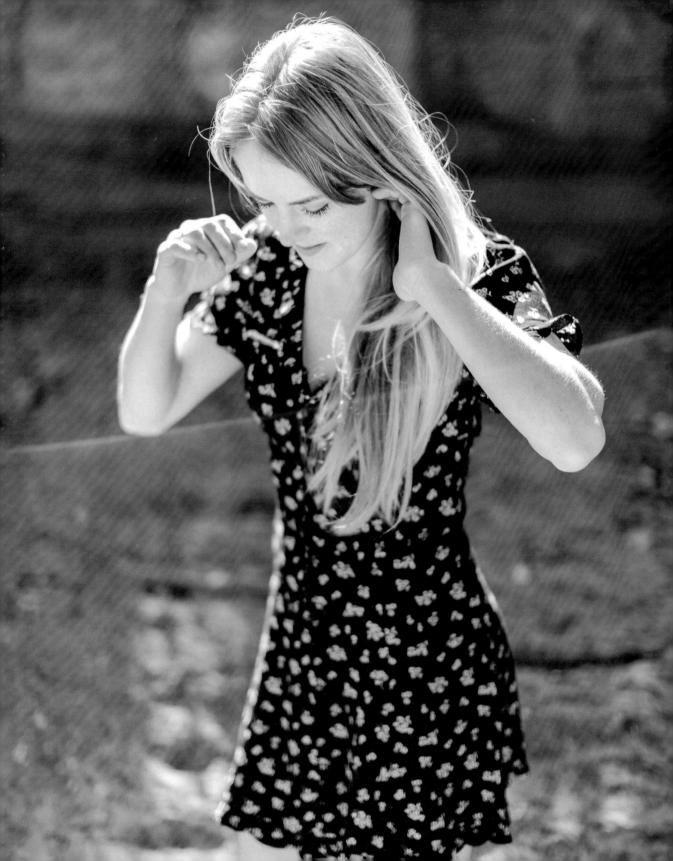

GETTING HERE

I spent half my life feeling less than. Feeling that I was lacking, whether in physical beauty, talent, intelligence, or creativity, I never felt like I could "measure up." This feeling of not enough sent me on a quest—I wanted to eat perfect, I wanted to look perfect, dress right, talk right, be in the "right" circles . . . I wanted so badly to accept myself, but I had put so many unattainable stipulations on the goal that it was unreachable in its format. I couldn't see my innate beauty, I couldn't grasp my (our) divine perfection. Conceptually I knew that "perfect" (in physical and mental form) wasn't something that was possible, but I still expected this perfection from myself. It took a lot of painful experiences, a lot of hungry days, many sleepless nights, sad relationship ends, maxed-out credit cards, shelves and shelves of self-help and diet books. It took many burned bridges and left me grieving, sometimes hardly breathing, with a broken heart and what felt like a million more issues. When you're lying on the ground like I was, it can seem incredibly hopeless. It can feel like nothing can breathe life into you, nothing can lift you out. The beauty of all of this is my quest for perfection led me to some pretty amazing messes. Messes that I wouldn't wish on anyone, but am overwhelmingly grateful for. My "issues" have been incredible teachers and have helped me transform what once was a scared little girl into really grateful and confident woman. In this book, I'm striving to share some of my most important lessons and some of the key practices that really helped me drop the facade and switch the direction of my journey. This book is written with deep love and appreciation for you, for your journey, and for your messes.

This is not a normal recipe book. Though it is filled with delicious and healing recipes, the focuses is on integrating all parts of ourselves, our bodies, our minds, our hearts and spirit. You'll be introduced to recipes, rituals, routines, and processes that supported me in becoming the most authentic and grounded version of myself. By making the recipes and following the rituals provided, you'll be playing with new ways of thinking while being supported in deepening your relationship with your full self.

I wrote this book to share with you what's been working for me. I also wrote it for me—I need this book! I need these reminders, these recipes, these rituals. I need consistency in holding myself and reminders of what we truly are. I want to continue a life that is infused with passion, I want to keep my kitchen filled with plant-inspired goodness, I want to care for my body with revitalizing rituals and holistic health modalities, I want to deepen my awareness and continue to use healing energetic practices, I need this book. I wrote it for me, for you, for all of us. Every single one of these pages comes from my heart with much love and healing energy. We really are all in this together. It's amazing what our bodies and hearts can do when we give them the opportunity to heal. Whatever it is that you are struggling with in life, whether it's in body, mind, or spirit, my deepest wish is that you find peace in knowing you are at the right place at the right time. I'm so glad this book found its way into your hands.

FOOD, HURT, AND HEALING

My experience with food has been one of deep healing and total rejuvenation on a mental, physical, and spiritual level. As a teenager and young adult, I struggled with disordered eating and low self-esteem. This is an all-too-common theme among many of us women. Like I shared in the introduction of this book, I was striving for perfection. Striving for something that actually we all already are, but I was seeing it one-dimensionally. I was seeing perfection from the eye of the old paradigm. I was seeing perfection as the cover of *Cosmo*, as the Barbie, the perfect body, the perfect face. I wasn't privy to the fact that the perfection I was really seeking lived within in me. I didn't know that by tapping into that essence I would feel more beautiful and radiant than I could ever have imagined. I heard the concepts such as inner beauty and the radiant feminine talked about by my mother here and there, but it didn't stick. It just felt like something older women spoke of. And in true honesty, the search for this external perfection seemed more exciting to me at the time. It seemed more glamorous than the search for spiritual understanding and inner beauty. But I can tell you now, it was not glamorous. Not in any way. I was bulimic—never being able to hold a meal down, feeling sick with myself, not worthy of being full. I was depressed, I was careless with my body, I was careless with my heart. It was not pretty. It was far from glamorous. It was tragic.

It took me until I was twenty-three to really grasp that something wasn't okay. Something deep was off, and I knew in my heart that I needed attention in another way. My mother always sent me books and set me up with intensive self-help

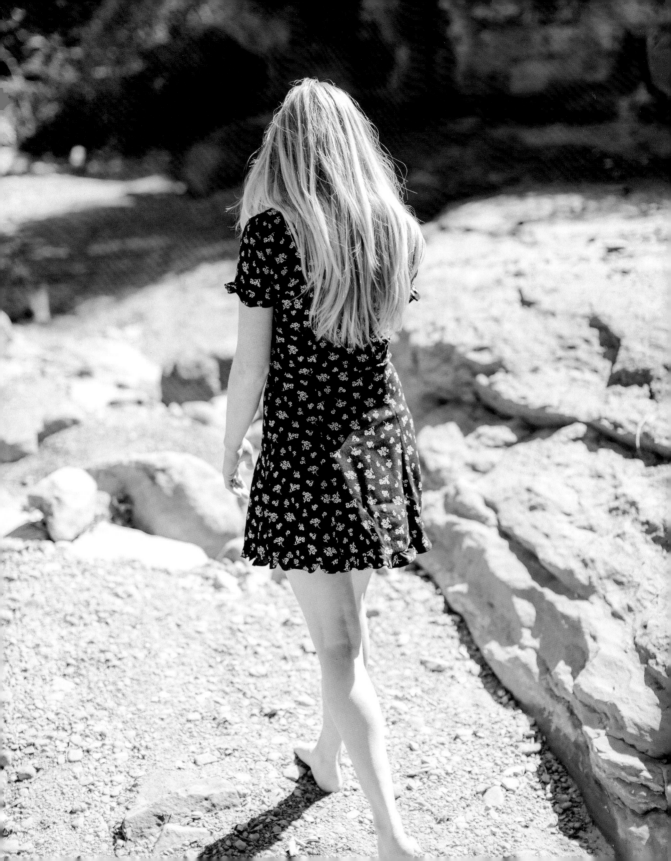

workshops and therapy sessions of one kind or another, hoping that I would at some point click back into my true essence. As a mother myself, I can't imagine the pain she went through seeing me live my life with such self-hatred. In 2009 I was living in San Francisco, in a little apartment in the Richmond, I remember finally picking up a book that had been sitting in my room for a while, *The Presence Process* by Michael Brown. That day was the beginning of my return to my self. *The Presence Process* along with Marianne Williamson's *Return to Love* were two of my guiding lights out of my unintegrated life and into a new way of living in the world.

Once I started reading these books, things changed quickly. I was finally ready for the shift. I was so low, so down, and so full of hate. I hated my body, hated my voice, my face, my life. I hated everything. I was in despair. I was at my lowest moment. There was nowhere but up or all the way down. Reading these books brought me out of my selfishness and reminded me that there is so much more, that we are so much more. Depression, in the way I was experiencing it, was somewhat selfish. My whole world was about me, what I wanted, what I needed. I never considered anyone else. Just me. How isolating. It was by remembering that it's *we* not *I*, that I finally broke me out of it. I remember the day I felt alive again. That morning I began a two-week juice fast, I meditated, took a walk to just enjoy nature, I quit drinking, I let go of the friends that were no longer serving me, and just focused on my well-being. By doing this, I became so much more in touch with others, so much more aware of others and so much more grateful. It turns out I really wasn't searching for perfection after all. Discovering a path toward self-love was the remedy. It was incredible. I felt new life breathed into me. I felt motivated, healthy, and hopeful for the first time in years. I began the processes of dumping my cultural beliefs of who and what I should be and began my journey to finding what I was without my "story."

Throughout this journey, food was always a big issue for me. It was filled with deep pain and it was shameful. I think that's why so much of my focus in the world now is based around food. I really needed to heal that relationship. I needed to bring healthy options into the world. I needed to create a safe place for myself to continue to heal. Historically, food is tied to the goddess—in the ancient times, crops and farming always needed to be blessed by the goddess, by the radiant feminine. The women would bless the men before they would hunt, the women were the sparks needed to bring food into the world and into the homes. It's interesting to me that nowadays food holds so much pain for women. The thing that we once had so much power over now holds power over us. I feel as though there is a spell that needs to be broken. A curse that needs to be lifted. This can only happen when more and more of us wake up to our truth and real beauty, wake up the fact that we are so powerful and magnificent. Wake up to the fact that we are sisters, not enemies, and what's mine is yours in the end. My story is still unfolding, this book and these words are healing me. Thank you for taking the journey with me.

IT'S A JOURNEY

Self-love is a journey, it is not a destination. We have been conditioned for so long to pick ourselves apart, disregard our true perfection, and seek flaws. This work of loving yourself is not easy. It's often really painful to find love in what we have deemed so unlovable. We all come into this world the same way, innocent, pure, and ready to give and receive love. The world is not always pretty, and our lessons are not always easy, but we are not alone. My story may be similar to yours, or maybe there are at least some themes within it that resonate with you. The main thing I really wanted to share is we all mess up. We all go through rough and rocky times, we all do things that our society labels as shameful, but what's really important is that we don't buy into that shame. I bought into for so many years and all it did was keep me down. Once I began to share more openly about my past struggles with eating disorders, alcohol, relationships, and self-concept I began to hear so many other women's stories. What struck me is how many of us share similar paths and how many of us feel so alone.

I feel so incredibly grateful for all my challenges. They have helped me birth my passions and have given me the opportunity to share my experiences in hopes of helping others find their healing journey. I wouldn't be writing this book if it weren't for my challenges; they've given me the confidence. I wouldn't have written *Raw and Radiant*, I wouldn't have opened my juice bar concepts, I wouldn't have known how to share.

My hope is that this book supports you to make the changes you're striving for in your diet, but really more in your life. I hope you find inspiration beyond the food, beyond the recipes, beyond the surface. My wish is for you to tap in fully to your own intuitive sense and begin creating recipes that will continue to heal your body, heart, and mind. You are a witch doctor, you are filled with secret ingredients that only you can offer. My intention is to help you unlock all that radiance that is living right underneath the surface.

I hope that you stop and smell the flowers, dig your feet in the earth, plant your own garden, put the phone down, and really revel in the beauty of your body and this amazing Mother Earth. I hope you feel the power of your spirit and the heartbeat of nature. Let these beauties be what fuels your life, let these gifts guide you into becoming a woman who knows her worth and walks in her power.

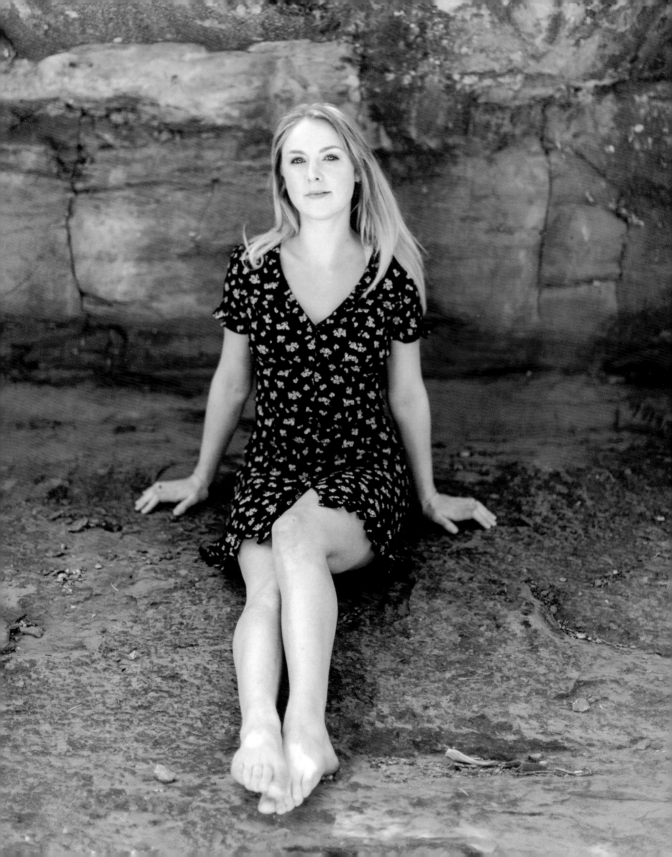

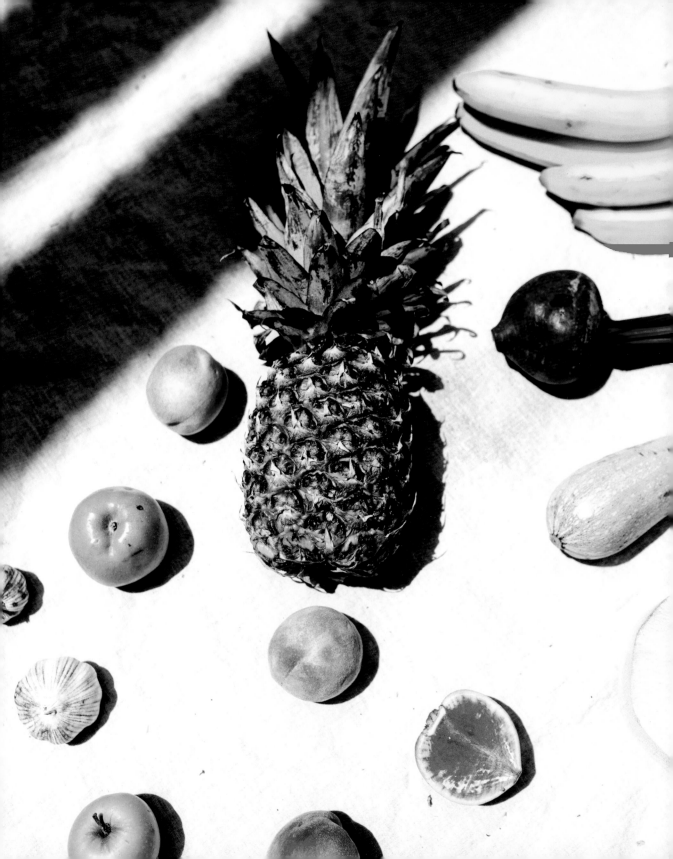

TIPS FOR USING THIS BOOK

This book can be used in many different ways—you can use it as a reference for times when you're needing a little extra support, you can follow the guidelines to a tee, or you can just find recipes that excite you! Whatever feels right.

It's divided into five sections: Inner Work, Beauty, Motherhood, Cleansing, and Food. My intention is for you to use this book as an ongoing resource for mind, body, and spirit wellness. I have a few tips before you get started that I feel will support you.

1. Commitment is everything. Your willingness to commit and follow through are what will make your life actually radiant. The tips here can only support you once you've made the commitment to love yourself. It's not easy—but it's so worth it. I hope you'll dig deep and harness all your light.

2. Small changes have big effects. Starting small with one or two of my suggestions will be the best way to make changes in your life. Pick one healing method or teacher to look into and pick one routine to support you daily. Maybe integrate a few of the recipes into your daily life. Don't let the bulk of the information overwhelm you.

3. Set intentions, not goals. Danielle Laporte, author of *The Desire Map*, has a method I love. She asks, "How do you want to feel?" versus "What do I want to get?" How do you want to feel? Set intentions for how you want to feel and start working toward the feeling rather than the "Goal."

4. What is your *why*? A wonderful question to ask when you're looking to commit to a change in any area of life. Why am I wanting to change? Is it because of external influence or is it a deep calling from within? When your why is coming from a deep authentic place, you're likely to really do some amazing work and be divinely led to what will heal and inspire you within this book and far beyond.

5. Progress versus Perfection. Be mindful of how you are gauging your "success." It's not about perfection, it's about making strides each day that support your deepest needs.

Feed yourself first, emotionally, physically, and spiritually, and then you'll have so much to offer to those you love. Unconditional self-care is an act of kindness to the world—and self-love is a lifestyle that you deserve.

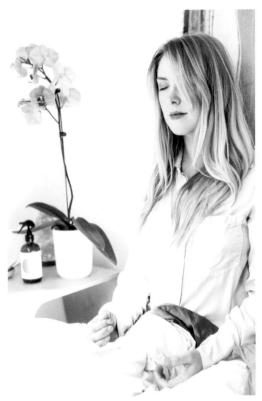

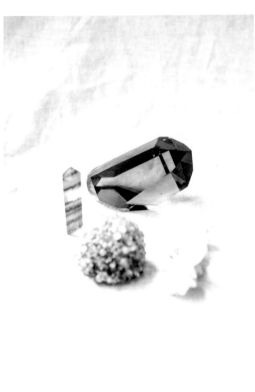

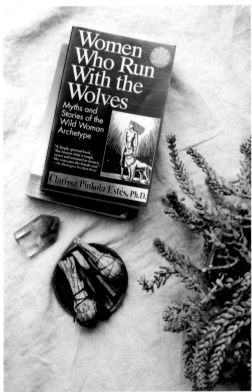

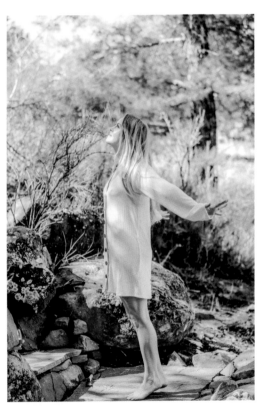

ON INNER WORK

THE CREDO OF BODY, MIND + SOUL WELLNESS

These are a collection of ideas and suggestions that were (and are) very helpful for me. As you'll hear me repeat in this book, pick and choose! Don't try to do everything at once. Find one thing you resonate with and give it a go. Then after integrating that into your life, pick another. Slow and steady is what keeps us balanced and on the path. This isn't about achieving, it's about soul work, and soul work has no time line.

FINE-TUNE YOUR INTUITION

Many of us have silenced our intuition, shutting it out and opting not to listen. Listening to what I like to call the *still small voice* that lives inside each of us is often our saving grace and way out of unhappy or "stuck" situations. Your intuition can serve you on many levels, and as a woman in the world, I think it's absolutely mandatory to exercise this blessing of a muscle. Honing your intuition (gut feeling) can help you in finding the right foods for your body, support you in healing ailments, mothering, relationships of all kinds, and navigating difficult life choices. We all have this deep knowing, but we've been somewhat conditioned by society to stop listening. Listen up, it's powerful when you begin to trust your body's communication systems.

I found that to reconnect to my intuition I had to stop all media for a while. I didn't listen to the radio, I didn't watch television or any movies, and I limited social media time. I needed time to really feel what was real in me and not the outside influence of others. After a couple months of this, my gut instinct was so strong and my confidence was soaring. I actually still practice this—I'm incredibly choosy about what I feed my eyes, my ears, and my body, because it all matters. Try a practice run! Do three days of no outside influence and watch what starts to surface.

EAT CLOSE TO THE EARTH

I believe eating foods that are as close to the earth as possible is one of the healthiest things you can do for your body. The absolute best is when you have your own organic garden that you can pick from. Even if that's just starting with some simple, easy-to-grow herbs in your window. Second best is shopping at your local farmers' markets and buying directly from farmers. Knowing where your food comes from and getting it while it's still vibrating and alive is a big part of getting all the nutrients that create health and beauty. Lastly, buying organic and biodynamic foods from your local health food store. Make sure everything looks alive. We are what we eat!

GRATITUDE

I know that this is a very commonly used term, but it doesn't diminish the beauty of the word and its meaning. Something I do daily to help create more upflow in my life is taking inventory of the positive around me. That can look like noticing beautiful art, or a gorgeous flower or the sun peeking through the clouds in a glorious way, or a sweet cuddle from my kiddo. It doesn't always look like gratitude for specific things in life, it can just be gratitude for a moment or even a feeling. This practice has brought so much happiness to me in a simple and easy way.

EMBRACE YOUR FEMININE AND MASCULINE ENERGIES

We each hold both masculine and feminine energies within us no matter our sex or gender identity. When we get imbalanced and fall too far into one way of being, we can become out of sync with our bodies and even unhealthy. If you resonate as primarily feminine but you find that the world (job, partner, roles you play) are continually forcing you into

your masculine, you'll become out of sorts and your root chakra begins to close up and even turn off. This can result in low energy, low sex drive, frequently getting sick, or feeling drained. You may find that you don't feel creative or driven by life. As I write this, I'm personally working with rebalancing my feminine. For the past five years I've been go, go, go, starting and running my businesses, working on a product line, writing my book *Raw and Radiant*, and raising my son while trying to balance a relationship. I relied on my masculine to drive these things. I fell into the trap of doing without balancing my self-care and female goddess energy. Thankfully I've come across some amazing healers and used many of these modalities and rituals to get myself back in sync. I'm still a work in progress, but I'm deeply enjoying connecting with my feminine parts and getting back into balance with myself.

GET CURIOUS

Nothing can ever change when you're just doing the same thing you've always done; you'll always get the same results. Change requires curiosity, intrigue, and honest self-evaluation. A clear choice to change is needed before you can shift your life, health, and body into a healthier state of being. Get curious about what will help you make the change, get curious about the things in this book, and get curious about what's driving you. Trying on a few different ways of living to see what feels good for you is something I encourage you to try. I definitely stay curious in my life and never set myself into stone. I'm open and willing to try new things and experiment with new ways of thinking and living. I'm also always asking why, why do I do this, why do I want this? Getting curious helps lead to clarity.

GO INTO THE DARK

It's always good to remember that contrary to what it might seem, often the darkest points in health (and life) can be the most amazing catalyst to lasting changes if we allow them to be. It often takes something pretty dark or drastic to shake us up and move us into change. This isn't true for everyone, but it certainly was true for me. By simply allowing yourself to be where you are and noticing all that surfaces for you, you can start with the work of soul alchemy. When you find yourself feeling really low, miserable, and depressed, don't try to push yourself into a different state; instead, try just validating your feelings and really letting yourself feel all the darkness that surfaces, remembering that you are made of light, so there is no way

this *feeling* can take over you. Check out page 279 for some wonderful books that have helped many with navigating this aspect of health.

When I go through dark times now in my life, I recognize that they are fleeting moments. I value the "discomforts" that stir within me, because they show me where I need to spend more time. They lead me to the areas within myself that still need attention. When I allow myself to be in the "dark" without judgment or fear of getting stuck in it, I am able to shine the light on these aspects of myself and move through the feelings for good.

STAY THE COURSE

Long-term health, wellness, and happiness don't happen overnight, but one simple choice to start does set you on the course. It's important to stick to it—we can get very discouraged if we don't see immediate change, but remember that even if it's not seen right away there are shifts happening that will benefit you for your entire life. Stay the course, pick yourself up when you fall down, and use your willpower. There is nothing as important in this life as your health and vitality. If you choose to try a new diet tweak or ritual, give it at least three months to integrate into your life.

CREATE THE SPACE

Creating a space that is conducive to taking care of yourself is one of the major keys to really sticking to it. This means creating the space in your home, your kitchen, your work, and in your heart. Decluttering, letting go of clothes, décor, and food items that no longer inspire you or make you feel good is a great place to start. Take one room at a time and really feel into what is serving you. Sometimes it can be really hard to let go of things even if we never use them. This year I did a massive letting go of household items—it was hard at times to let go of things I felt attached to, but I'm so happy I did. My home feels so much more relaxed, and I do half the amount of cleaning! It left me feeling clean and clear on many levels and able to give attention to my passions and family instead of constantly feeling bogged down by cleaning up.

MOVE YOUR BODY

Moving your body daily in some way is a very important. Your body thrives when it moves. having a daily exercise routine helps to flush stuck energy, cleanses your lymph, and creates an opportunity for change. I often get my greatest inspirations on my morning walks. You don't have to do intense workouts, a 30-minute walk or simple yoga routine is wonderful and can be incredibly uplifting on many levels.

UNPLUG + TUNE IN

Put the phone down, turn off the computer, take off your watch. For two reasons: the radiation and electromagnetic energy that comes from these gadgets is incredibly harmful for your body, especially when we are on or literally wearing them all day. They are all addicting. We can't get really deep into ourselves and our health when we are continually distracted and comparing ourselves to lives on Instagram! Unplug, feel yourself, feel your life. Use these things as tools, not as a clutch for insecurities and undercurrent addictions.

MASTER THE ART OF PAUSING

Something that has been subtle in action but radical in its payout for me is pausing. Simply pausing before I respond. Pausing before I say something, pausing before I hit send. Pausing. Just taking a moment to examine my thoughts, my intentions, and my undercurrent energies. Some questions I ask myself: Is it really important for me to say this right now? Will it help or hinder the situation? Is this something I would be okay with sharing with everyone? Am I coming from a place of love or jealousy? Am I grounded in my body? Am I triggered? Asking these questions has really helped me come from a place of love and authenticity versus my shadow side. Just bringing awareness to this has been amazing for my relationships with others and with myself.

IT'S MORE THAN THE EXTERNAL

Eating clean and taking care of your body on an external level are very important practices. You've got an amazing temple to care for! But beauty is so much more than what we eat. Real, lasting beauty comes from the inside and radiates out, it's not something you can buy or eat. I've found that the most beautiful women I know are the ones that have been through it, that have really, really been tested and have decided to rise. They own their stuff, they don't claim to be perfect, they embrace their flaws and strive for a radiance that is eternal.

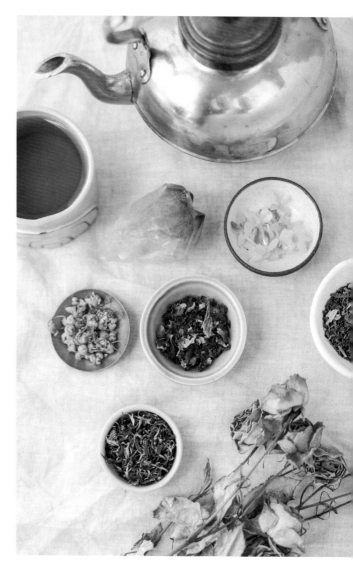

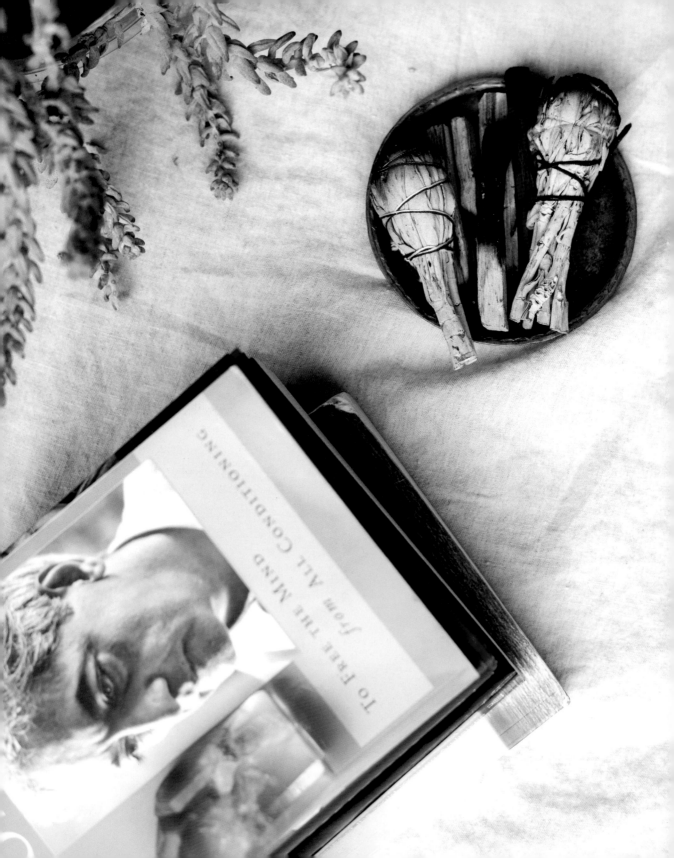

TO FREE THE MIND *from* ALL CONDITIONING

HEALING METHODS, MODALITIES + GUIDES

I've gathered some of the methods, ideas, and teachers that have been helping me in this journey toward self-love to share with you. Pick and choose! It's not about achieving perfection, it's about finding peace in the moment and supporting your deepest heart. Some may resonate, some may not. You'll gravitate toward what's right for you at this time.

ALONENESS

There is a difference between loneliness and aloneness. It's just like the difference between selfish and self-love. Sitting in stillness, deciding to be in *aloneness* is a really beautiful and healing state; whereas loneliness just keeps you in your head. I found that by deciding to not have outside influence and being with myself, I felt a kind of freedom and space for deep reflection. I was able to see clearer, to make decisions based on what was real for my heart and not just my mind or by those around me. Making time to just be alone can be a wonderful beginning to a healthier relationship with yourself.

SHADOW WORK

Shadow work is something that my mom spoke about for years, but took a while for me to latch on to. It deals with integrating the dark parts of ourselves and transforming negative emotions. I recommend picking up the books *Owning Your Own Shadow* by Robert A. Johnson, *Bringing Your Shadow Out of the Dark* by Robert Augustus Masters, and *Shadow Work* by Dr. Michael Ruth.

REPARENTING

Reparenting has been such a blessing for me. My history is rocky when it comes to a stable family environment. My biological father was schizophrenic and committed suicide when I was young, my godfather (who I consider my dad) was an alcoholic, my stepfather whom I loved dearly left with no warning. My mom was fearful and likely felt alone in it all. I've been dealing with these abandonments for years. I've tried a lot of different methods, took courses, went to workshops, read the books, but the thing that for me was most effective and heart healing was reparenting. John Bradshaw is one of my favorite authors on this subject. His lectures and books on healing shame and working with the inner child are really accessible and not intimidating at all; he's very human and grounded. His work has been major for me. Lacy Phillips of *To Be Magnetic* has created a wonderful online course called Unblocked that is a great place to start with this concept if it's new for you.

THE WORK BY BYRON KATIE

The Work by Byron Katie has become pretty popular over the last couple years—her work was and is still a refuge for me. The Work is a very simple method to help us take responsibility for our thoughts and current life state. She helped me to see myself clearly and also to see the humor and lightness of it all.

THE PRESENCE PROCESS BY MICHAEL BROWN

This process was my introduction to breath work and my reentry back into my real life. I put this in here because it truly helped me shift my disordered eating and start to really see things from a broader view. I recommend this book to anyone and everyone. I'm still reading it! I cycle it all the time.

INTEGRATE

The most important one! Many of us have a lot of methods and modalities, we've read hundreds of books, we go to the workshops, we follow the accounts, but we fail to integrate. We fail to actually use the methods. We just keep accumulating new methods hoping that that will heal our hearts, that going to the lectures will somehow raise our vibration, and maybe it does, for a moment, but without doing the work and really following though, you'll never grab what you're reaching for. This was one of the hardest lessons for me. I had so many tools, I just failed to use them. Once I actually began to use the tools, things changed.

KRISHNAMURTI

One of my favorite authors and speakers. J. Krishnamurti supports us in questioning all authority and dropping all the facades. Sounds hard because it is hard. Krishnamurti's lessons are not for the faint of heart, because they really call you to look closely at your mind, your ego, your life, your conditionings, and to honestly witness them. When you get quiet and observe all the ways your mind works, the patterns, the shadows, the tricks, you'll be more able to witness it all without action. Just a soft watching without judgment. I often have to read or listen to only a small amount of his work and then really take time to digest it. Sometimes I'll just read one passage over and over until I feel I really understand the intention behind it. I love listening to his lectures, hearing him speak his words is very powerful for me. I also love spending time at the PepperTree Retreat (Krishnamurti's old home) in Ojai, California. The library and educational center are amazing, as is the lush property.

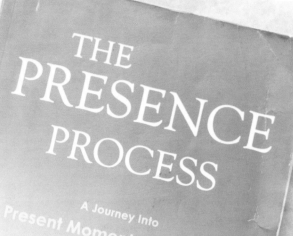

THE
PRESENCE
PROCESS

A Journey Into
Present Moment Awareness

Revised Edition

MICHAEL
BROWN

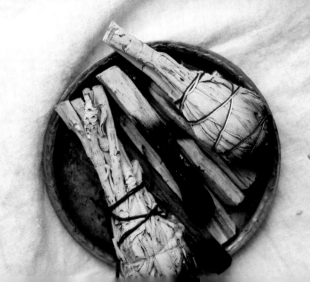

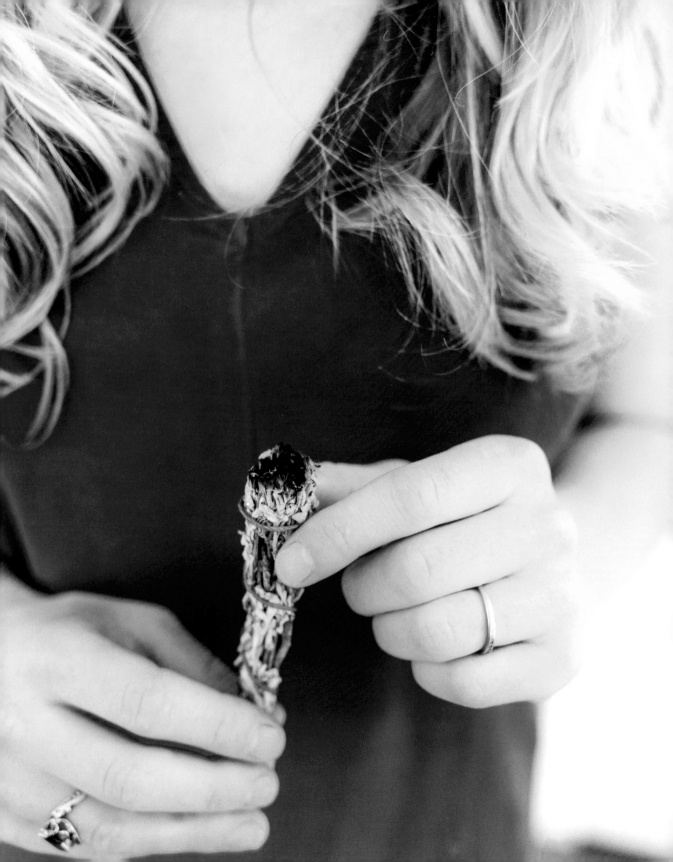

MANTRAS + THE POWER
OF INTERRUPTING PATTERNS

I'm adding this part in because it has recently come back into my life in a big way. During the day we think a lot. We say a lot to ourselves inwardly. Unfortunately for most of us, the things we say and our mental chatter is typically not very positive. To make matters worse, we often unknowingly repeat these things to ourselves over and over throughout the day. These thoughts become patterns, and often manifest into our reality. There has been much flack for mantas lately and I understand why. Just saying over and over to yourself, "I'm beautiful, worthy, and capable," won't do much of anything if you don't really feel it within. Well I agree, you need to feel what you're saying in order for it to really do deep work, but I also see (and have experienced) how shifting the mental chatter to a positive over a negative has intrinsic value. What I've found is that by using a mantra, I begin to shift the mental talk. Every time I catch myself in the normal guilt, shame, or fear talk, I stop it. I replace it with the positive mantra. At first it might not ring true, and my ego will reject it. But if I'm consistent and use it daily, I start to weave a new pattern—one of self-love and respect. I think the ultimate goal is to have a deep knowing of our worth, but because we are such wounded creatures, we need rehab. That's what mantras are for me. A path back to the realness and wholeness that we are. Baby steps.

Something I have found is that saying the exact opposite of what my mind is saying helps break the pattern. For example, if I'm caught in a pattern of saying, "I'm bad with money," then I change that to "I'm great with money"—again I am hyper-aware that just saying something doesn't make it true, but interrupting the pattern can be helpful. I've also found that because I don't want to be a fraud, I make moves when I begin saying something like "I'm great with money." If I'm saying that every day, several times a day, it's going to help keep me from making frivolous purchases and maybe support me in starting to really invest in learning about how to be great with money! I feel that it's really all about coming from a place of love versus fear. Changing our mental chatter can really help with this.

When it comes to mantras, I believe they are highly personal. I don't think there is as much strength when you're just repeating words that someone gives you; this really needs to come from you, thus I won't be providing any mantras in this section, but do encourage you to play around with creating your own.

MEDITATION

Meditation is something that I always have found amazingly helpful. When I was seventeen, I was gifted a guided meditation CD (before the online apps and resources) and I remember how much it grounded me and opened my heart. I have gone back and forth with using meditation since then. When I look back and feel into the times of my life where I was most happy and feeling divinely connected, meditation played a part. There are still times in my life today when I am not meditating, but I feel it instantly whenever I choose to start. Meditation can be as easy as setting aside five minutes a day for breathing. It doesn't need to be extravagant. It can be whatever you need it to be. I have been using an app called "Insight Timer" which gives access to free guided meditations as well as courses.

ASKING WHY

If you don't ask questions and ponder why things are the way they are, how will you know what is true for you?

There is a book called *Start with Why* by Simon Sinek. It's about leadership and authentic business and making a human connection. In the book, Simon states that it is not what you do, but why you do it that makes something successful. This simple leadership philosophy carries over in to our personal lives in a big way.

"It's not what you do, it's why you do it"

Many of us just function out of habit. We wake up, check our phones, have our coffee, respond to emails, pour the cereal, pack the lunch, carpool the kids, and off to work. But we forget that fundamental question . . . Why? Part of living a vibrant life is starting with why. For everything you do, ask the question, "why?" Why, is a powerful question that will help you get to know yourself on a deeper level and see where some of your past may be interfering with your present. I believe that questioning all authorities (even our own inner "authority") is a wonderful path to freedom and to learning what really pleases us. When we begin to really ask the "Why" and do our own inner research, we're free to create rituals that really serve us and climb up the right ladder, so to speak. This how we begin to break the norm and determine what success and happiness really look like for us as individuals.

When we start to ask why, we can see our social traps and see the things we are genuinely doing because it touches our souls. We can see where we are conforming and where we are expanding. I know when I started to ask why, a lot shifted. My relationships, my diet, my total way of living. I started to make choices based on what I truly wanted my life to be versus just living the social norms.

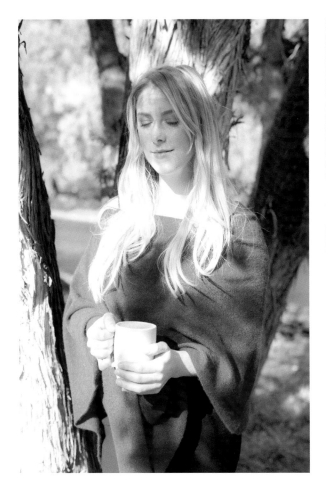
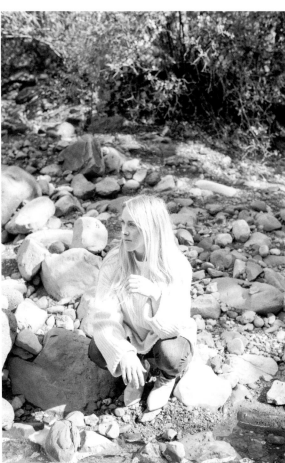

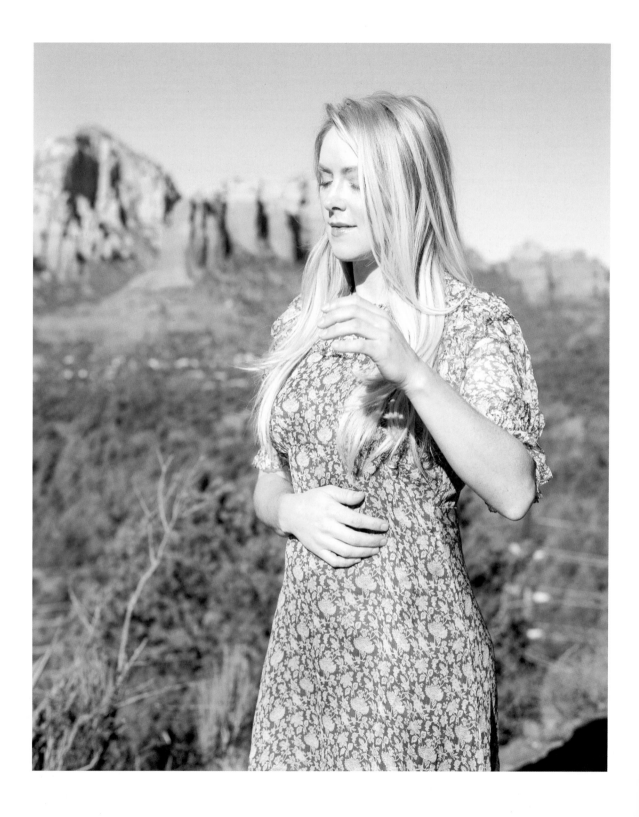

CALLING ON THE GODDESS

I have to admit, it's taken me a long time to get comfortable with the word "goddess." Not because I don't think a goddess is something absolutely worthy, just because of my conditioning around the word. Maybe you even feel that little tinge of aversion within you right now. Try saying "god" out loud—that feels normal, right? A word like "goddess" is so absolutely powerful! And it should be used.

Until more recently, I didn't use the word "goddess," and I thought it was hokey how people used it. It felt foreign and even forced. . . . But I realize that that was because I didn't feel powerful as a woman, I felt like I was at the whims of my emotions, I felt scared to step out on my own, I felt shame, I felt anything but goddess-like. I felt unworthy of using the word, so of course it didn't feel comfortable.

I did realize that I wanted my son to have a "balanced" feel for God, not just a masculine essence, but the feminine as well. When we would do our little prayers or blessings I would say, "thank you to Father God and Mother Goddess," which is where I first noticed my hesitation to use the word. But I went with it anyway. Because I felt so

much aversion to it, I decided I needed to start studying goddesses a little more so I could fully understand what I was saying and calling upon. I started by buying every book on goddesses and amazing women who embodied the archetypes that I could get my hands on (which I share on page 279). It clicked for me. We aren't comfortable with the word "goddess," because she's been cast out. She was removed, killed, and subjugated to a minimal role in our society. Someone knew that when a woman knows her true worth and power, all bets are off, and she'll rule the world. So they shoved her to the back and tried to burn her legend, but through myth and stories and amazing women, she lives on. There are five main things that I learned from my studies of the goddess that I want to pass on to you. I do hope that you take a deeper look into some of the amazing books and resources on pages 277–279.

MOTHER OF THE UNIVERSE

Everything that is anything was birthed from a woman. Our Paleolithic ancestors understood this. Tribes dancing in birthing caves with goddess mother figurines, praising the almighty woman. Asking for her blessing, praising her like we should.

Becoming comfortable with our maternal nature is something we can all benefit from. Even if you have no dreams of becoming a mother, the maternal aspects of *you* want to be used. First off, it's important to take a look at what a healthy mother is. Many of us didn't get the blessing of have a fully functional and healthy mother; the lineage of the pained women is long.

A healthy mother is strong but kind, tender at just the right moments, and forceful when she needs it. She's a warrior, a defender, a lover, a warm embrace. She's comfort, she rational, yet aware of the divine. Take a moment to write down what a healthy mother means to you. Once you get these down on paper, circle the ones you feel are most important to your life. Which of these attributes do you need most? Do you need more comforting? Do you need protection? Fierceness? Become these things for yourself and you'll be able to offer these to others without your life force being drained.

We as women give so much of ourselves just like our Mother Earth, but it is of the upmost importance that you first give to yourself so that you can sustain the others. Mother yourself first and you'll be one happy woman.

MASTER OF THE MIND + EMOTIONS

Women by nature are feelers—we feel everything. We sense, we pick up on, we intuit. We have big feelings, and it's easy to act on them. Something that we can learn from early goddesses and powerful women of today is to pause. There is so much beauty in your emotions. So much wisdom, but often that wisdom gets lost or misinterpreted when we act without evaluation. Something that will help you harness your power and build up your inner strength is mastering these emotions, not changing them or avoiding them but using them and performing alchemy. This is what really brings thoughts into tangible things. This practice can be a really easy or a really hard one; it just depends on your readiness to commit. When you're ready to witness yourself and watch your mind with compassion and caring, you'll thrive.

Next time you have a strong emotion, whether it be anger at your partner, coworker, or family member, or lust, or sadness, take a minute to pause. This would be the time when you might normally send a text message you instantly regret. Pause. Watch your mind, see how it twists the emotion. See how it turns it into something that isn't true? *They did this to me, they don't understand me, they hurt me, they don't want me, they used me . . .* watch these thoughts. Ask "is it really true?" Watch the story you tell yourself. You can talk to them: "I see you." "Thank you for the lesson," "You can go now." Sometimes I visualize a trash can and I see myself throwing the thought away. It's not about avoiding the feeling, it's about detaching from the thought so that you can really feel the emotion behind it. When we place blame we miss out on awesome opportunity to feel and to eventually heal.

Once you drop the thought, you get to really feel it. That tight feeling in your chest, the bowling ball in your stomach, that ache in your throat. Feel it. Let it be there, don't try to change it, don't try to move it. It's your power! You don't want to sabotage this beauty of a thing. This pain is your salvation. Dance it, sing it, paint it, bring it to life; it wants to be born. Channel your pain, channel your emotions. They want you to use them, to witness them, to accept them, and to transform them. Do this one thing, and your life will forever change. You've integrated a part of yourself that been aching for you.

POWER FROM WITHIN

At any moment it could all disappear. Your house, your car, your clothes, your things. They could go at any time. Hold that for a minute. Who would you be without your "stuff"? This is a powerful question because so many of us are identified with our life belongings. Our fancy car, our designer clothing. Reality check: They mean nothing. But you mean everything. At the end of our lives, we will not be counting our diamonds, we'll be counting our blessings and the love of our family and dear ones.

Developing a strong sense of self that is based on your inner beauty (far beyond looks) and strength is the ultimate goddess move. Take a moment to take inner stock by answering some of these questions.

What do you value?
How are you living that is not in alignment with your heart's values?
How can you make a change today to better live your truth?
How do you treat people?
How do you treat yourself?
How do you want to be treated?
Are you aware of the difference between your mind and your true self?
Can you watch your thoughts and stay unattached?

Some of these questions are hard ones that really challenge us to make major changes or at least bring awareness to our current state. If you want to go deeper into this, I recommend picking up a book by J. Krishnamurti or Eckhart Tolle, anyone will do! Their ability to get right to it and pose important questions can be a powerful foundation for creating a strong sense of self as well as witnessing our all oneness.

LOVER OF THE ARTS

Women need outlets. Outlets for the many feelings that swirl around within us. When not given an opportunity to free themselves, these feelings can wreak havoc and become volatile. They can act out as depression, anxiety, addiction, self-sabotage, over-giving . . . But when you funnel your feelings into creative endeavors, magic happens.

As I'm writing this, my heart is split in half. My life as I know it is changing, and it puts a tight rope around my heart. My throat feels clenched, and my stomach is nauseous. It's raw, it's real, it's painful. Writing this, sharing on these pages is medicine. It provides a small fracture where some of the intense feelings can drip out. When I'm done here, I'll sit at the piano and wail some sad songs, I'll indulge my pain. Music, art, writing: They all support the release of suffering and help it to transform.

Goddesses have always been masters of the arts. It's not only incredibly attractive to indulge your passions but also therapeutic as you read above. Take time for yourself, beautiful woman, enjoy the gifts of the feminine.

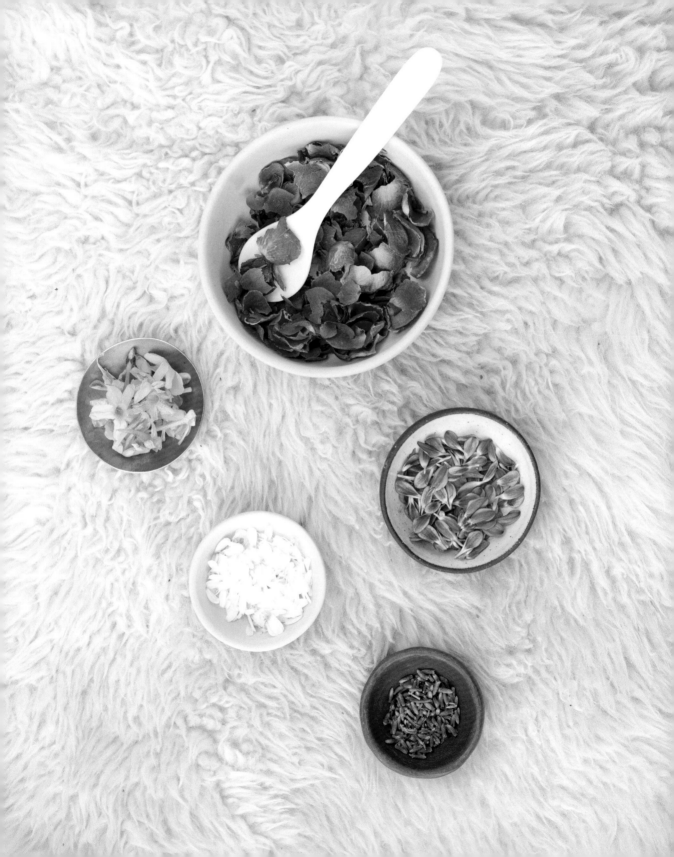

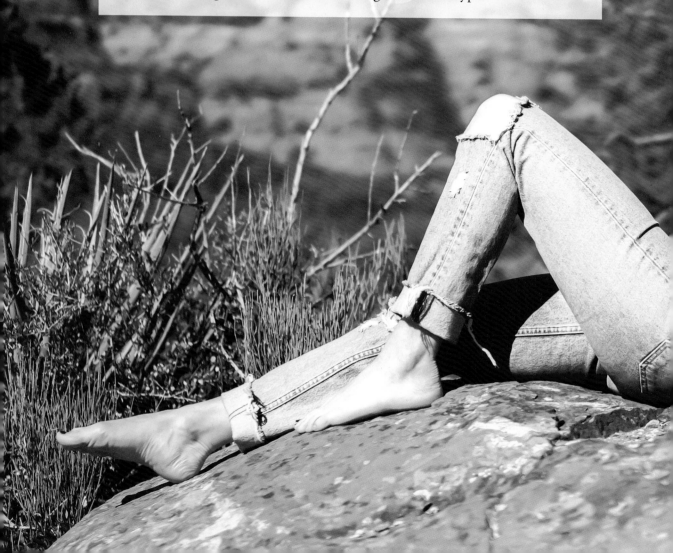

SACRED SEDUCTRESS

The goddess archetype was never just a beauty, she was a powerful sexual being. Take Inanna, Aphrodite (in her pre-patriarchal role), Lilith—they all were lusty but what fueled the fire of their sex appeal was all the other attributes discussed above. Without a keen mind, cultivated talents, internal power, deep caring, the ability to access empathy, a sense of how to use their mothering instincts, their sex appeal would be dormant. These goddesses were the full package. Something to remember here is that physical beauty is not one of the five goddess pillars. Though external beauty is always a great foot in the door, it is not enduring. What we learn from the goddess archetypes and the women who have embodied them is that cultivating a rich personality and a strong sense of self is where the magic lies. Our society is obsessed with the outward appearance, but those who fall prey to this short-lived game are always left in a deep pit with not much assistance in getting out.

Sex is so much more than the act. The energy you carry within yourself and about yourself are a major part of real sex appeal. Seduction is not about lingerie, though it can be fun to play that role. Seduction is about energy and depth. It's about giving of one's self and receiving gifts from another. It's a powerful tool when used with concision, and a reckless, empty one when used for the wrong reasons. A real goddess knows the difference.

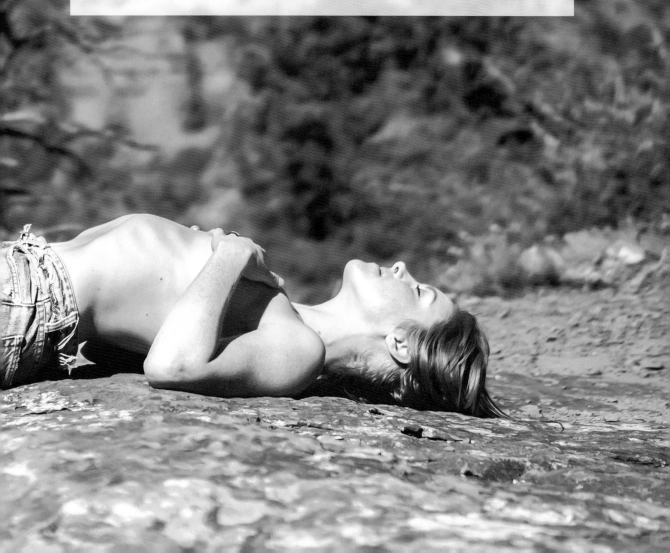

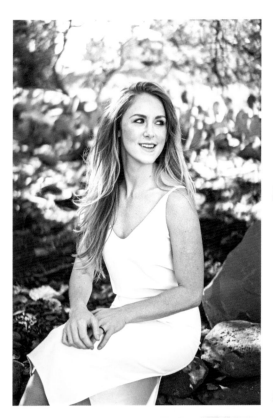
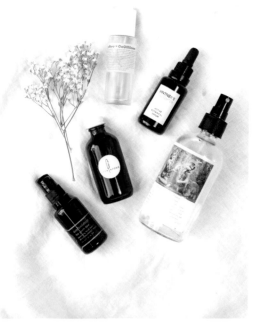
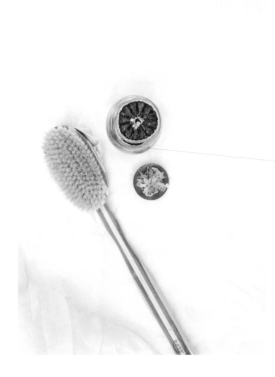
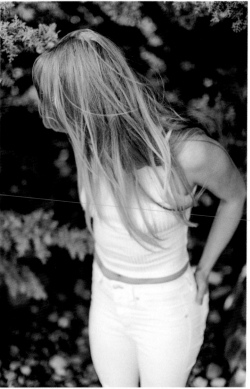

ON BEAUTY

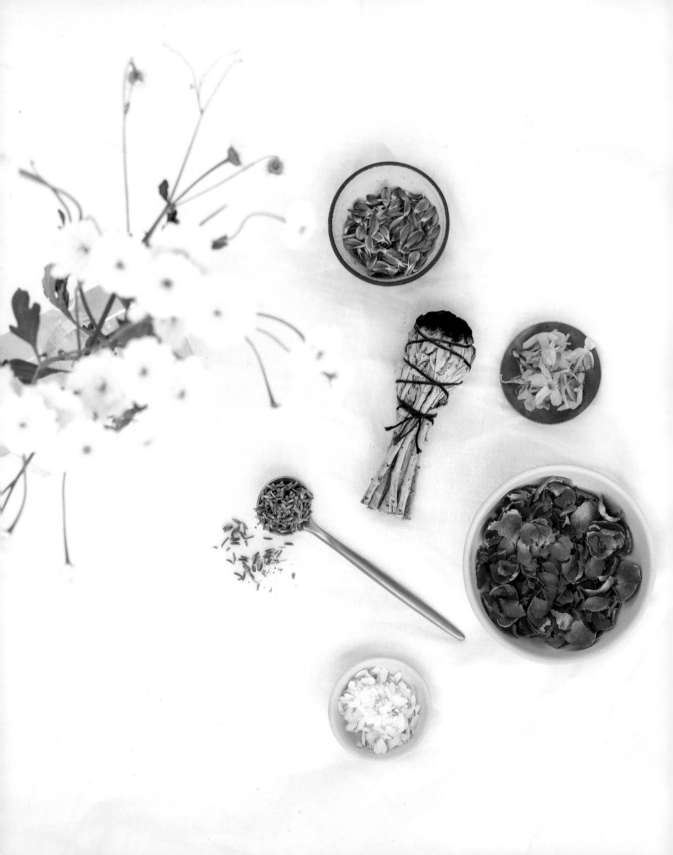

HOLISTIC BEAUTY

In this section I'll be sharing some of my favorite beauty recipes. These are simple recipes and rituals you can make and do yourself at home. Some of these rituals are ancient; some are newer personal creations. Take what you love and embellish with your own personal flair.

An important truth I wanted to share in this book is that beauty is truly so much more than skin deep. You can be the most beautiful woman in the world externally, but if you're not tapped into the deep river that runs within you, no one will see your actual radiance. Radiance and Beauty are two very different things. Radiance is something that is felt, it's something that you can't buy, it's cultivated and it's a real gift. I truly believe that by digging deep into the dirt and the pain of our lives, detangling the knots and shedding the layers, we tap into real beauty that radiates and transcends.

Caring for ourselves and nurturing our bodies with these sweet beauty rituals is one way we can really start to make space for getting to know ourselves. Take time with yourself, spend time admiring your body and all it does for you. Create time and space to adore yourself. Beauty routines can be a very touching form of self-love.

Our skin is the largest organ in our body. It takes in everything. I like to think of it as our outside digestive system. Whatever we put on it, will eventually be in us. That's why I'm so big into using great water filters and only clean beauty products (see more on page 277). There are so many chemicals and toxins in our water and products. These chemicals can really negatively affect your hormones, detox organs, thyroid, and lymphs. It's very important to be aware of ingredients and toxins. The recipes that follow are all natural and plant-based, with no dangerous chemicals or fillers. I do suggest that you patch test each first.

SKIN MASKS + SCRUBS

FOUNTAIN OF YOUTH MASK

This is a classic new age mask. It's clay and apple cider vinegar, that's it. Both these ingredients can be found online or at your local natural foods store. I used this mask all through high school and still use it today. It's great for minimizing pores and clearing out impurities, it always leaves my skin feeling great and looking supersmooth. It can be a bit drying, which is good if you have oily or combination skin. Just make sure to moisturize well afterward. You can add your favorite essential oil into this mask to cut the strong smell of the vinegar.

Makes 1 mask

---

1 teaspoon apple cider vinegar
1 tablespoon French clay or
  bentonite clay
1–2 tablespoons water

Whip all ingredients together with a fork until creamy. Use a brush or clean hands to apply to your face and neck. Leave on until dry and then remove with a warm washcloth.

HONEY ROSE MASK

I love this mask. It's antibacterial, helps minimize pores (thanks to the French clay), and smells divine. It's great for all skin types and really easy to make. I love Mountain Rose Herbs (www.mountainroseherbs.com) for all apothecary needs. They carry high-end organic essential oils, clays, herbs, and even jars for storing your creations.

Makes 1 mask

3–5 drops rose essential oil
1 tablespoon raw honey
1 tablespoon French clay
1 tablespoon water

Whip together all ingredients with a fork until creamy. Use a brush or clean hands to apply to your face and neck. Leave on for up to 1 hour and then remove with a warm washcloth.

MATCHA MASK

Matcha is my favorite superfood, the absolute ultimate beauty product both internally and externally. Double down and make the Matcha Latte on page 89 while enjoying this luxurious facial mask. The antioxidants in matcha are powerful for your skin. This mask is great for skin that tends to be a little on the oily side. It's also wonderful for around your moon cycle. It will calm any hormonal breakouts that may surface. You can find French clay online at www.mountainroseherbs.com or at your local natural foods store.

Makes 1 mask

---

1 teaspoon matcha powder
1 tablespoon raw honey
1 teaspoon French green clay

Whip all ingredients together with a fork until creamy. Use a brush or clean hands to apply to your face and neck. Leave on for up to 1 hour and then remove with a warm washcloth.

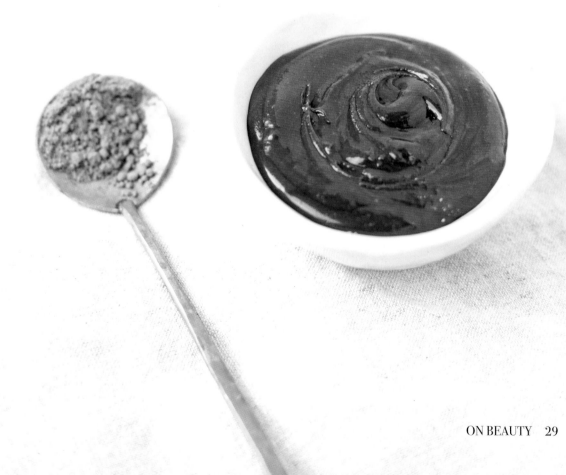

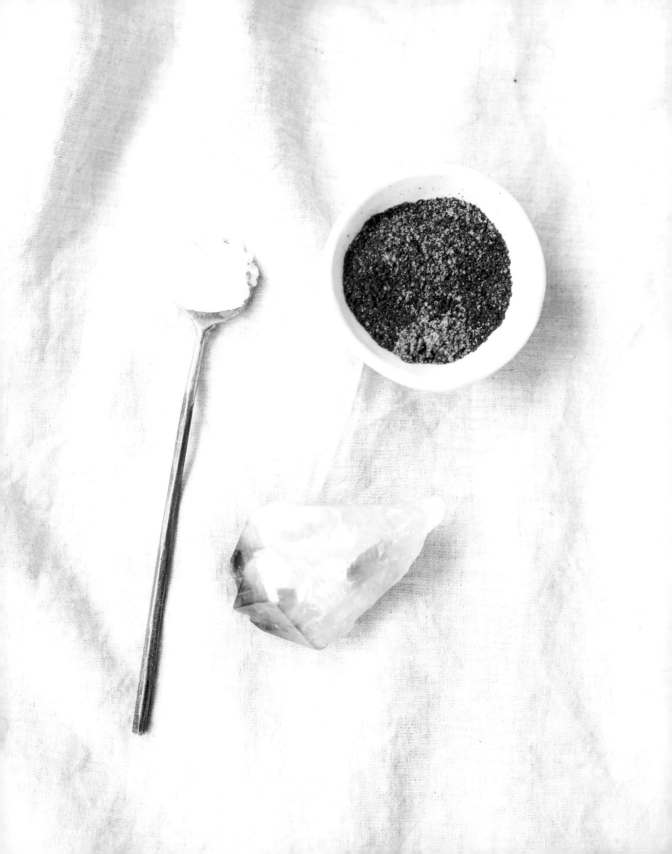

COFFEE BODY SCRUB

This is great for in the shower; it buffs off dry skin and leaves you glowing. I absolutely love the feel of my skin after this amazing scrub. Add any of your favorite essential oils in to customize it! Coffee scrubs have been known to help with cellulite and skin tone in general.

Makes enough for up to 4 uses

---

1 cup organic coffee grinds
½ cup brown sugar
¾ cup coconut oil
5 drops vanilla essential oil (www. bulkapothecary.com)

In a medium bowl, combine all ingredients. Mix together until well-combined; you may need to use your hands to get the grounds and the coconut oil mixed well. Store in a glass jar for up to 1 month.

SUGAR SUGAR BODY SCRUB

For the softest, most glowing skin all day long, try this in the morning for an all-over scrub. I even use it on my face! Great for elbows and knees or very dry patches. This scrub is perfect for everyday use.

Makes enough for up to 4 uses

---

3 cups organic cane sugar
½ cup brown sugar
10 drops lavender essential oil
6 drops neroli essential oil
3 drops rosemary essential oil
1 cup coconut oil

In a large metal bowl, combine sugars and essential oils. Melt coconut oil in a double boiler, then pour into the sugar and essential oil blend. Stir the mixture quickly. Put into your favorite sealable jar and cool. This scrub will keep for up to two months when stored in an airtight container.

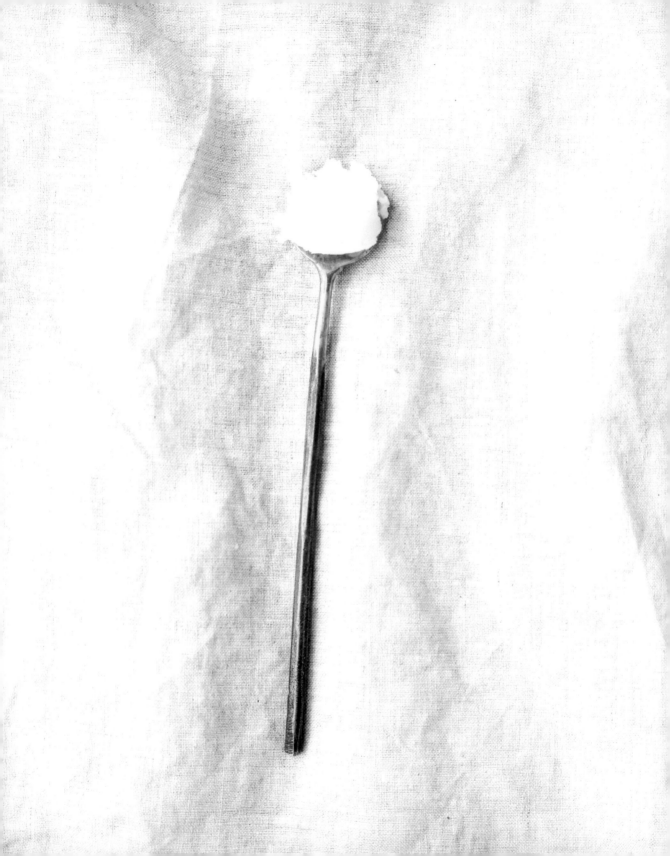

HAIR TREATMENTS

COCONUT OIL HAIR MASK

One of my longtime go-to hair repair treatments. Its literally as simple as slathering coconut oil all over your hair! I wanted to sex it up a little bit with some amazing essential oils. I love ylang-ylang and bergamot, also a little chamomile and jasmine. Coconut oil is known to help reduce hair breakage, prevent hair loss, and prevent protein loss. Coconut oil has lauric acid, which is a medium-chain fatty acid that makes coconut oil easier for the hair shaft to absorb. I suggest using this mask as a prewash treatment. You can also keep it on overnight for an extra deep hydrating mask.

Makes enough for 1 mask depending on hair length

½ cup coconut oil
3 drops ylang-ylang oil
3 drops bergamot oil
3 drops chamomile oil
3 drops jasmine oil

In medium-sized bowl, add all ingredients and use a whisk or fork to whip the mixture.

Massage into dry hair and wrap up in a small towel. Leave on from 15 minutes up to overnight for an even deeper moisturizing treatment. Rinse with shampoo and follow with your favorite conditioner.

AVOCADO LAVENDER HAIR MASK

I love this for moist shiny hair. The smell of the apple cider vinegar is strong, but this really works miracles for shine. Adding the chamomile essential oil makes it a luxurious treatment.

Makes enough for 1 mask

Flesh of 1 large avocado,
  whipped
1 tablespoon apple cider vinegar
2 tablespoons coconut oil
2–3 drops chamomile essential
  oil
5–8 drops lavender essential oil

In medium-sized bowl, add all ingredients and use a whisk or fork to whip the mixture.

Massage into dry hair and wrap up in a small towel. Leave on from 15 minutes up to overnight for an even deeper moisturizing treatment. Rinse with shampoo and follow with your favorite conditioner.

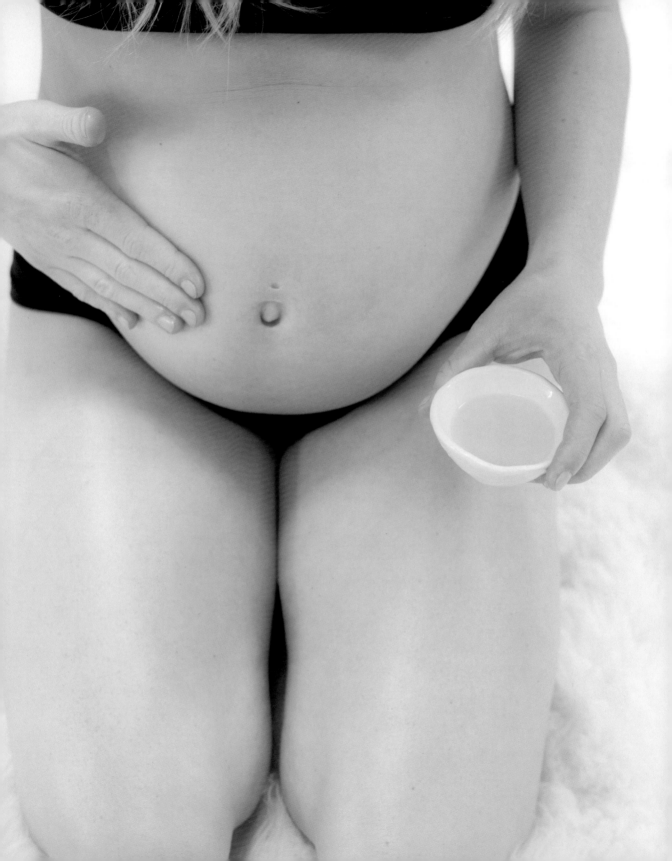

MOISTURIZERS

MOTHERHOOD OIL

This is my go-to oil for rubbing on my tummy and thighs when pregnant. With both pregnancies I've started as soon as I knew I was pregnant. If you're are planning on becoming pregnant, begin now! It helps your skin stretch with ease.

Makes roughly 2 cups

1 cup sweet almond oil
1 cup vitamin E oil
20 drops lavender oil
10 drops neroli oil
5 drops frankincense oil
3 drops patchouli oil
5 drops bitter orange oil

In medium size bowl, use a whisk or fork to combine all ingredients. Then use a funnel to pour into your favorite glass bottle. Use roughly 3 tablespoons daily on tummy, back, and thighs.

VENUS OIL

Love yourself up with this special healing oil. Great for both body and face and safe for everyday use. Prickly pear seed oil is wonderful for its antiaging effects. You can find it online at www.bulkapothecary.com or in specialty shops.

Makes roughly ¾ cup

½ cup jojoba oil
¼ cup vitamin E oil
2 tablespoons prickly pear seed oil
8 drops ylang-ylang oil
8 drops cinnamon oil
8 drops lavender oil

In medium size bowl, use a whisk or fork to combine all oils together. Pour into your favorite glass bottle with a pump. You can order these online or fine at specialty shops. This oil can be used daily and keeps for up to 5 months when stored correctly.

MANGO BODY BUTTER

This is a very thick and luxurious body butter, great for post-pool or in the very dry months of summertime. Add a little water to your hand as you apply the butter. This will help your body absorb the moisture. The blend of mango butter, coconut oil, and cacao butter is so thick and hydrating, you'll be glowing from head to toe.

Makes roughly 1½ cups

---

1 cup mango butter
(www.bulkapothecary.com)
¼ cup coconut oil
¼ cup cacao butter
5 drops palo santo essential oil
5 drops clary sage essential oil
5 drops orange blossom
  essential oil

On the stove top, slowly heat mango butter, coconut oil, and cacao butter on low until melted. Once the butters and coconut oil are a liquid, add the essential oils and whisk. Play with these essential oils! Add whatever you love. Then package into a glass widemouthed jar. This body butter keeps well at room temperature.

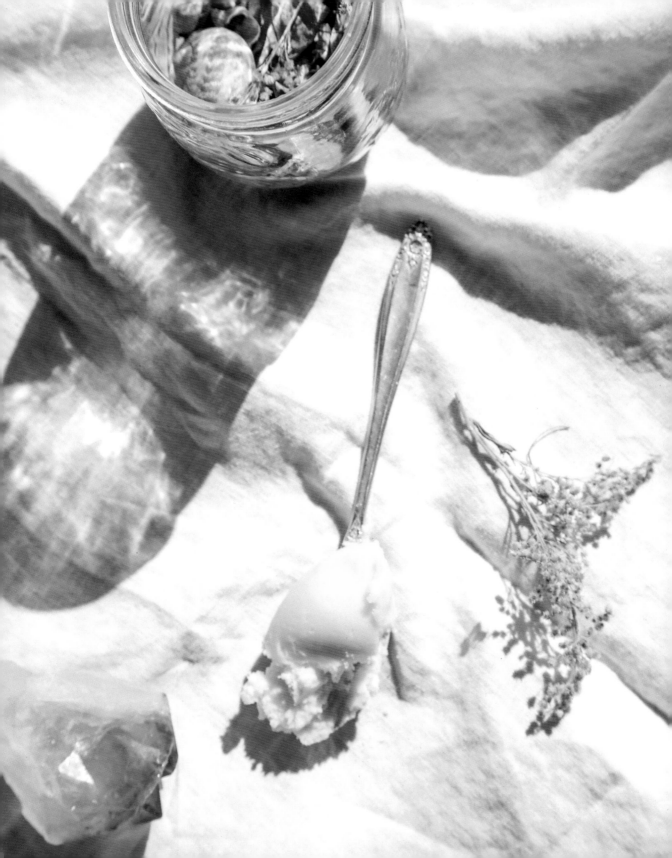

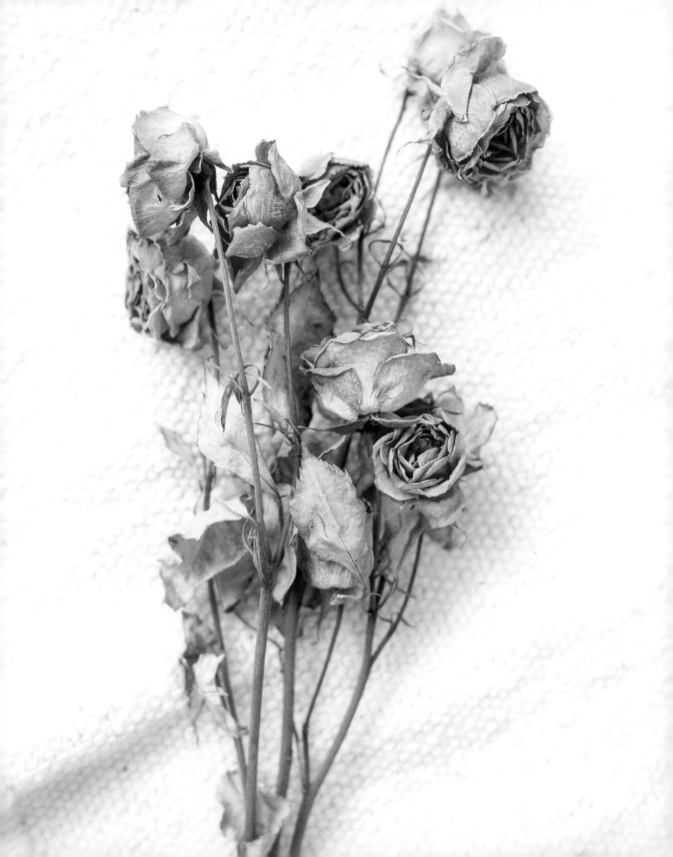

BATH SALTS + SOAKS

ROSE PETAL SOAK

There is something so beautiful and sacred about roses and water. Cleansing, healing, and indulgent in the most wonderful way.

Makes 1 Bath

---

1 cup Epsom salt
10 drops rose essential oil
1 cup rose petals, fresh or dried

Fill a bath with hot water, and pour in salts, followed by the essential oil and rose petals. Put on your favorite relaxing music, light a candle, and totally relax.

BAKING SODA BATH

Baking soda is known to help reduce CO_2, return our pH to alkaline, and neutralize radiation. If you have a headache or lung issues, I always suggest a baking soda soak. I do this soak for my son Henry. It's totally safe for kiddos.

Makes 1 Bath

---

2 (16-ounce) containers baking soda

Fill a bath with hot water, then pour in the baking soda. Immerse yourself completely. After a few minutes, stand up and pat down your body with a towel, then submerge your body again. Do this a few times for the best results.

SORE MUSCLE SOAK

This soak helps with sore muscles and also helps neutralize radiation in the body, win-win!

Makes 1 Bath

---

1 cup Epsom salt
½ cup apple cider vinegar
1 (16-ounce) container baking soda
12 drops lavender oil

Fill a bath with hot water, pour in the salts, vinegar, baking soda, and essential oil. Immerse yourself completely. Enjoy the feel of the hot water on your skin and let your body fully relax.

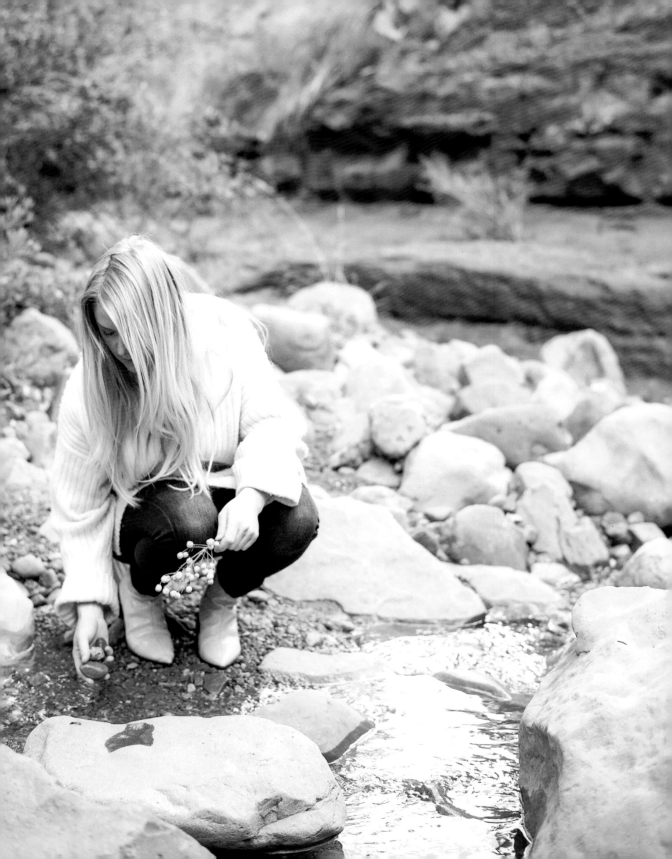

HORMONES

Skin quality, weight, and emotional stability go hand in hand with hormones, but hormones are not often talked about. If your thyroid is off, your weight will likely be affected, if your estrogen is high, you likely have breakouts, if your progesterone is too low, you may be bloated all the time. These things are important to address because it could be a small fix that helps you feel lovelier and just overall healthier! One thing I've been really loving is cycle syncing—eating, moving, and living by my moon cycle. Alisa Vitti is the author of *WomanCode* and has an amazing App called Flo that supports woman in syncing their cycles and fixing their hormone issues naturally. Check out her app and book. She's helped thousands of women, including me! I've laid out some basics below to get you started but to get the full picture get Alisa's book.

THE FOUR PHASES OF YOUR CYCLE

FOLLICULAR: 7–10 DAYS

The follicular phase is a higher-energy time. When it comes to workouts, dancing, lots of good cardio, or hiking are all great options. You want to be moving your body and supporting your system in moving out toxins though sweating. Enjoy fresh foods that support your body in elimination. Kimchi and sauerkraut are especially wonderful during this phase, as well as lots of salads, lean protein, sprouted grains, and seeds.

OVULATION: 3–5 DAYS

This is a great time to move your body! Your body is feeling all the feels and is full of sexual energy. This is a perfect time for high-intensity workouts, think Soul Cycle, hot yoga, or other fun high-intensity training. Your body is at its peak when it comes to energy, and you're likely feeling really strong. Support your body by loading up on raw food! Fruits, veggies, nuts, and seeds. Light fare is best for this time.

LUTEAL: 10–14 DAYS

Alisa recommends that the first part of this week is dedicated to slow strength training or intense yoga. Scaling back later in the week when you're closer to your cycle is the best; your energy needs to be directed inward to support a happy moontime. Your body is working hard and needs the slower pace and extra healthy carbs. Walking, Pilates, and relaxing yin yoga are great options. Food-wise, filling up on roasted root veggies (especially yams!) and greens is best. Keep it low sugar and drink lots of water!

MENSTRUAL: 3–7 DAYS

During your cycle, it's more about inward focus and calm action. Taking time to support your body with meditation, gentle yoga, walking, or slow mat Pilates. Eat food high in minerals such as nori, seaweed, and kelp to help replace any lost nutrients. Adding in healthy protein and fats while still keeping it fairly low glycemic will serve you best.

HORMONE HACKS

LIGHTS OUT

Shut the lights out and use candles after 6:00 p.m. I resisted this at first, but now I love it. I read by candlelight and love the cozy feeling. You can also purchase orange lightbulbs for your home that block blue light, but I find it a little more romantic to do candles. Most homes have LEDs now, and these are incredibly toxic to our sensitive systems. Using candles, orange bulbs, or great blue-blocker glasses will really support your hormonal health.

LIMITING SCREEN TIME

In the evening and early morning is hard for me because I often have to work at night or in the morning before my family is up. I have blue-blocker glasses and a filter on my computer but when I can, I try to have all electronics off by the time the sun goes down and not turn them on again until the sun has fully come up. The blue light affects your hormones and circadian rhythms. If you find yourself randomly waking up at 2:00 a.m., you are probably getting too much blue light. Dr. Sara Gottfried, author of *Younger*, has a wonderful seven-week protocol for hacking hormones and genetics and she focuses a lot on blue light and screen time. I definitely suggest reading one or all of her books!

MEDITATE

Meditation and relaxation can help calm the adrenals (hormone power station) and support your body in fully relaxing. This in turn supports good sleep and healthy regeneration. Meditation has so many powerful healing effects. Even just five minutes a day will support your hormonal health.

EAT BEFORE CAFFEINE

Eating before you drink any kind of caffeine is a radical shift I made in support of my hormones. Also making the change from high-mold coffee to either Bulletproof or an organic, single-origin, locally roasted brand can be helpful as well. Even better is switching from coffee to matcha or organic black tea. I like to rotate these! Caffeine is fine to indulge in, but making sure to have a meal before you do coffee or tea can really be healing for your hormones.

TOUCH THE EARTH

In the morning, walk outside and let your bare feet touch the earth for 5 minutes. This is called Earthing or Grounding. The basic principles of this is that you will be exchanging the Earth's electrons. By going out into the morning light and touching the Earth you are sending your body the signal that it is morning and time to produce specific hormones that you need during the day.

LOW WI-FI

Turn your phone on airplane mode at night and always keep it away from your body! Consider unplugging your router at night to minimize radiation from Wi-Fi. I use a wired system at my house. There is no need to have it on while you are sleeping; this is your time for regenerating. Let your home be sanctuary for regeneration in the evening.

NO PLASTIC WATER BOTTLES

The BPAs and phytoestrogens in these bottles can become big disrupters for your hormones. Opt for a glass or stainless-steel water bottle that you fill with filtered water.

CONSIDER NEW FORMS OF BIRTH CONTROL

I'll let the experts talk on this one, check out Alisa Vitti's book *WomanCode*.

LEAN ON NATURAL BEAUTY PRODUCTS

There are so many chemicals in most beauty products, and these chemicals can be dangerous for your health. You can find a list online at of the top concerning chemicals at www.safecosmetic.org See my list of clean beauty products on page 277.

DIG DEEPER

The Hormone Reset Diet and *Younger* by Sara Gottfried
WomanCode by Alisa Vitti
The Adrenal Thyroid Revolution by Aviva Romm

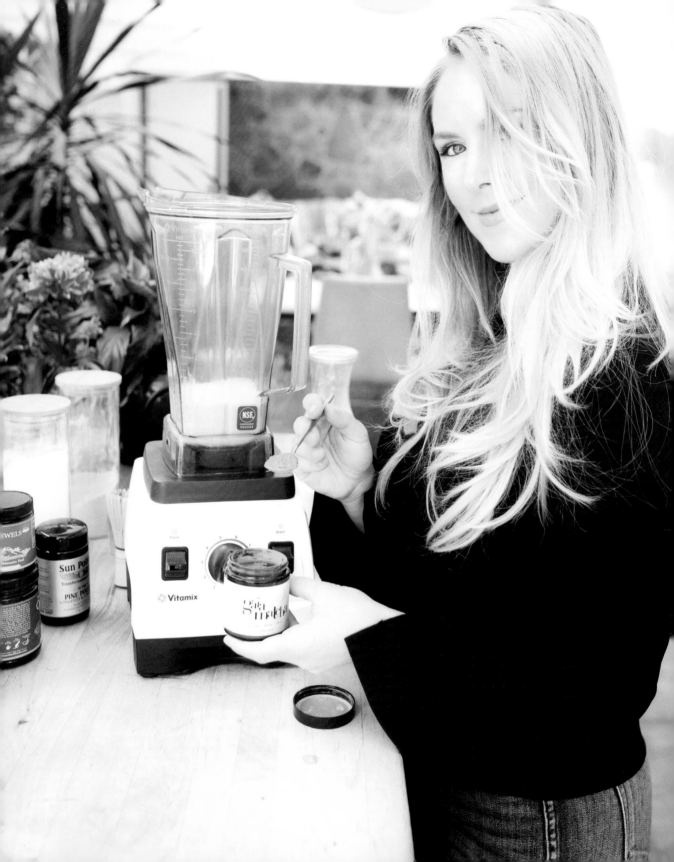

SELF-CARE RITUALS LIST

Healing rituals are vital to self-care. It's really about starting where you're at. Don't worry about adding all of these ideas into your life right now. Just do what you can, when you can. It's not about getting it "perfect" and doing everything, it's really about incorporating things into your life and morning that support you and make you feel good. You don't want to feel stressed about missing the morning routine steps! That's not the point. Just add what feels in flow and what you have time for. These are just suggestions based on rituals that have supported me—you'll find what works for you! This is something to turn to for inspiration. Routines are powerful; what we do daily starts to become a part of us. It's important to do things daily that support and nourish your body, heart, and mind.

DAILY

- Three-minute face washing to activate blood flow. Use a cream-based face wash in the winter and a liquid one in the summer.
- Cold shower in the morning.
- Exfoliate and drain your lymph by using a skin brush.
- Fifteen minutes of rebounding (jumping on a small trampoline) to your blood flowing and support your lymph drainage.
- Thirty to sixty minutes of exercise. If you're a woman, it's best to sync your cycle and workout. See page 41 for more on cycle syncing and its benefits.
- Upon rising, drink eight ounces of room-temperature water (cold water is stressful for the liver, and hot water kills naturally occurring enzymes) with one half lemon or lime squeezed into it. I opt for lime in the spring and summertime and lemon during the fall and winter seasons.
- Breath work such as Qigong or a simple practice of deep connected breathing.
- Herbal tonic or green juice and healthy breakfast (see page 135).
- Meditation or visualization (see page 14).
- Morning sunshine, best when in the nude!
- Nature, even if it's just taking your shoes off in the backyard.

WEEKLY

- Some form of bodywork weekly is worth its weight in gold. Taking time to really appreciate nature and love on your body. I love Alphabiotics, which is a very gentle adjustment for your brain and body. Massage is a great option, too. If you don't have the resources to outsource bodywork, self-massage is a beautiful form of self-care and deep loving—you can also ask your partner to help with this part of self-care. It can be a really sweet offering for both of you.
- Baking soda bath, for alkalizing the body and removing excess CO_2 (see page 39).
- Sauna or steam.
- Coconut or avocado hair mask (see page 33).
- Full body scrub (see page 31).
- Facial peel (I love the Juice Beauty brand).

MONTHLY

- Lymph drainage massage.
- Vitamin B_{12} shot (if vegan).
- Intervenes Glutathione.
- Acupuncture.
- Organic facial (you can do this at home too! Check out page 28 for mask and scrub recipes).
- Cryotherapy (you can also do this at home with an ice bath!).
- Chiropractic.

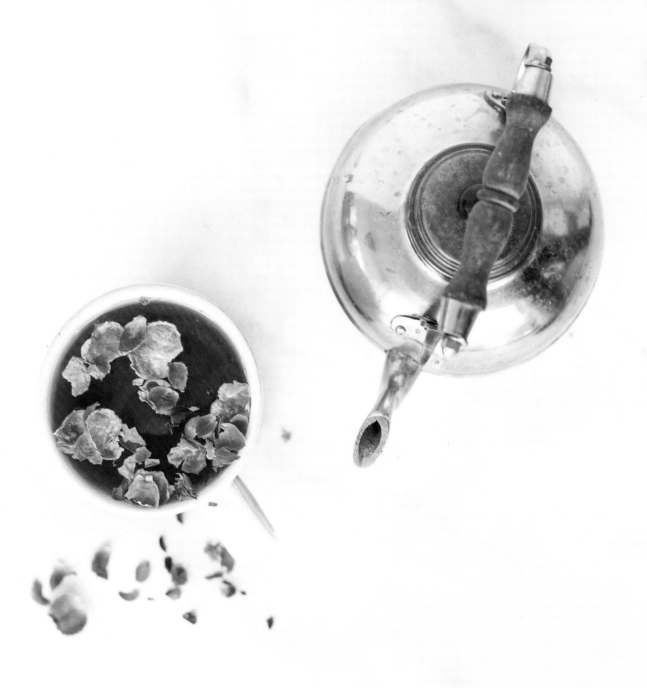

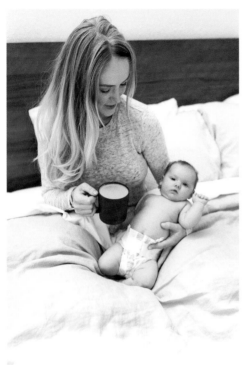
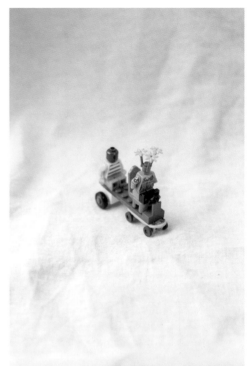
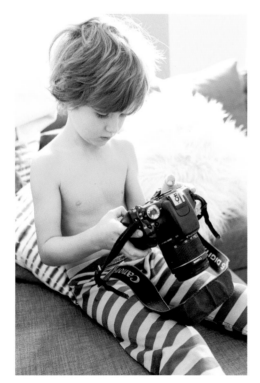
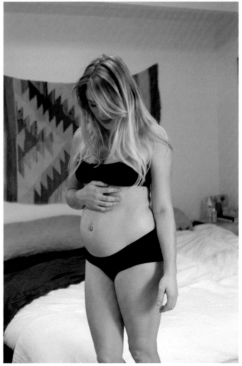

ON MOTHERHOOD

PREGNANCY

What a precious time. As I'm writing this, I'm seven months pregnant with my second child. It's been a completely different pregnancy than the first and I've already learned so much about the baby and myself. In this section I'll be making some offerings and bringing up some new ideas to consider. Pregnancy and child-rearing are so very personal, and each woman must follow her own instincts and inner voice. The best thing you can do is learn about different options and then make educated decisions based on what feels good for your heart and family. All I'm offering here are some different ideas to ponder on how to do things. It's incredibly important that you work with your trusted care provider to make decisions regarding the health of you and your baby; I'm sharing my experience as a mother and health coach, not as a pregnancy expert.

IN UTERO

What you consume both mentally, emotionally, and physically, are all making the fibers of your baby's being. If you're watching stressful TV, listening to scary news, and eating chocolate by the pound to try and sooth yourself, your baby is picking up on it. Just remember whatever you feel, baby feels, too. This is not to shame any mamas—we all go through incredibly stressful times, especially during pregnancy—this is just to remind us to tune in, turn off the news, take some breaths, and connect with the little one who is growing inside you. Everything you feel is okay, your baby chose you and signed up for it all, so don't feel guilt or shame if you've been stressed. This is just a gentle reminder to bring it on home

and give your sweet body and baby a little rest and relaxation. Deep breaths, warm baths, walks with your loved ones, healthy stews, and lots of water will all support you and your baby to melt into the moment.

WI-FI + RADIATION

This is often a controversial subject, but mainly because people don't like to change what is comfortable; we feel threatened by the things we don't understand. Our phones, our computers, routers, cars, smart meters, and smart homes all put off harmful radiation. Limiting the exposure to your body while pregnant (and after) is incredibly important. I see mamas with their phones tucked into their pants right where their growing baby is! I know if a mother knew the consequences of radiation from our gadgets, they would take major action. Nowadays in cities you'll find cell towers on schools, churches, and many government buildings. It can feel intimidating once you start to read the research and get educated on the facts. Our world is moving fast with tech, and there are a lot of benefits to that, but there are also drawbacks that we need to be aware of. There are so many ways to protect your family and growing baby from those harmful effects and still keep a normal life. These are my resources for education and protection. At our house we have dial-up, no Wi-Fi! If we need to turn it on for guests, we do have that option, but we don't use smart appliances, we turn off the Bluetooth and Wi-Fi in our cars, we leave our phones on airplane mode most of the time, and we don't let our children use the phones or tablets. These are just a few small things you can do to protect yourself and your family. It may seem extreme, but I urge you to dig a little deeper into the research and make a decision based on understanding.

NATURAL BIRTH

Birth is absolutely amazing, no matter what your scenario. The experience is crazy and wonderful! It changes you, it's a rebirth in a way, a coming into your own as a mother. Consciously choosing how you want your birth to go and not just relying on the "experts" to decide for you is important . . . while also being soft enough within your heart and mind to adjust to a birth that takes on a life of its own. We can plan for the "perfect" birth but God, spirit, universe, ultimately will take us on the ride we need. I believe that birth has been shown as a scary and painful experience, something to fear rather than to look forward to. There is absolutely a time and a place for medical interventions, but our bodies were built for natural birth, and this can often be the safest option. Let your love and deep knowing guide you, not your fear and imprints from society. Use your deep knowing and intuition along with educating yourself on all your options.

My son Henry was born at home. I was surrounded by loving, caring people, the light was low and warm, the bed was there waiting for me and my baby, the tub I birthed in was warm and supportive. It was an incredibly intense birth and it was incredibly beautiful. I labored for twelve hours and had back labor the entire time as Henry was posterior. I was massaged by my husband, supported to move into different positions that would help me ease the discomfort. I was in amazing hands. My midwife had been practicing for thirty years and was an expert. I felt safe and I trusted my body to do what it was made for! And it did. I wanted a home birth and I prepared for it for nine months. I was sure about it from the get-go and am so glad I had this experience. I also preregistered at the hospitals nearby and had a birth plan just in case the universe had other plans. Being prepared for all possibilities doesn't mean you're not trusting your body, it just means you're being smart.

Giving birth in a hospital is completely fine and can save lives—it's okay if hospital birth is your path or what needs to happen because of your circumstance, but going in knowing that you can have a say on many things is helpful, especially for a first time mama.

Some things to consider asking your doctor:
How long do they allow you to labor before inducing?
Are the drugs they offer drowsy?
How do the drugs affect the baby?
Can you have a doula with you?
What if you want to labor standing up or on all fours?
Is there a water birth option?

Do they give the baby right to you?
What is the policy on clamping the cord?
What is the reasoning for C-sections, vacuum, and forcep intervention?
How many people will be in the room?
What is the lighting like?

What is important to remember is you are the one who has to live with all the aftermath of birth. You have the power to decide how you want your birth to go and who you want there. There are many important decisions and you should feel what the right answers for you are.

MILK PRODUCTION
Breastfeeding is such a beautiful way to feed your baby. There is absolutely nothing better than your mama milk. There are a few things that can interfere with your milk production. If you start to notice that you're not producing, check these things: Are you using a pacifier? Drinking or smoking? Supplementing with a bottle? How is the baby latching? Not feeding enough? Not getting enough fluids? Working out too much? All these things can play into your milk supply dwindling. Check out La Leche League for more advanced support.

FOODS + HERBS THAT SUPPORT HEALTHY MILK FLOW

Alfalfa

Anise seeds

Apricots (fresh is best)

Barley grass shots or powder (add the powder to your smoothies!)

Coriander seeds

Dill

Fenugreek

Fennel

Flaxseed

Green juice galore (you really can't get too much)

Oats

Oat straw

Papaya

Red beets

Yams

SUPPLEMENTS

Calcium

Chlorella

DHA

Iodine

Krill oil

Magnesium

Methyl folate

Vitamin B

Vitamin B12

Vitamin C

Vitamin D3

Vitamin E

Vitamin K

Zinc

Please check with your medical care provider before ever trying new foods or supplements when pregnant.

FAVORITE PREGNANCY BOOKS + FILMS + SITES

The Business of Being Born by Ricki Lake and Abby Epstein
The Fourth Trimester by Kimberly Ann Johnson
Spiritual Midwifery by Ina May Gaskins
www.indiebirth.com
www.mamannatural.com

FAVORITE PREGNANCY FOODS + LIBATIONS

Chocolate Hazelnut Chia (page 153)
Classic Blueberry Muffins (page 239)
Date Shake (page 125)
Fennel tea
Ginger tea
Mint tea
Red raspberry tea
Savory Socca Pancake (page 141)
Stuffed yams (page 213)
Wheatgrass or barley grass shots or wheatgrass juice powder

PARENTING

Parenting has been my biggest teacher. It has taught me much about the capacity of the human heart to love. It's taught me about pure ecstatic joy, about deep pain, about my shortcomings, my breaking points, and the parts of my childhood that still need healing. It's taught me about what I value and it's taught me that I have so much still to learn. Parenting has been the single biggest learning experience of my life. It has led me to think that when we open ourselves up to the lessons of parenting and look at our children as not just small humans but our teachers, we open ourselves to an amazing journey. It doesn't mean we'll do everything right, it doesn't mean we won't mess up (a lot!), it just means that we are open to seeing ourselves clearly. Nothing is more powerful than clarity.

I debated on whether or not to include this section in this book—I'm not an expert, and I don't claim to have it all together in the parenting department, but I still felt that some of these topics are worth talking about and sharing. Maybe you resonate with a few ideas and words. For me, it's always been wonderful to hear other mothers share about their parenting journeys. We can learn so much from each other.

THE WORKING MOTHER

I remember the first year of my son's life. . . . We were a military family living in Encinitas, California, far from my family and friends, I only had one girlfriend, my husband literally worked from 5:00 a.m. to 7:00 p.m., and I was so lonely. I adored my son and did all I could to hold it together, but often I just felt desperate for adult connection and conversation. I had moments when I truly didn't think I could handle another moment of it. When he was nine months old, I started my business Local Juicery. I left California with Henry while my husband stayed behind for another year to finish up in the military. I worked my ass off to get my business off the ground, and my little guy suffered the consequences. I worked sometimes eighteen hours a day before I would see him. My mom would bring him to nurse at my shop. It was so hard. I think about going back and changing the way I did things, but it was what it needed to be for my learning and experience. We as women have hard decisions to make. We want families, but we also want to feel fulfilled creatively and professionally. Balancing parenting and work is incredibly challenging and there is absolutely no such thing as perfect, no matter what you choose.

What I've learned is that it's important to examine what success means to you. Is it monetary? Is it rewards and achievements? Is it freedom? What does it mean to *you*? Also ask yourself, "What's good enough?" Maybe you would like to bring in an extra hundred thousand a year, but maybe if you just shifted around a couple things in how your family lives, what you're bringing in now would be good enough. You could relax more in a simpler definition of success. It doesn't mean don't follow your passion, it just means enjoy the seasons of your life and your children while you can.

After opening my business, I was stressed to the max trying to make it work, take care of my little guy, be a wife, stay healthy, and make great dinners. I basically collapsed with adrenal fatigue about six months after opening. I had been living on coffee, waking up at 5:00 a.m. to go to the gym, nursing on demand, trying to learn how to run a business, and deal with the ups and downs of a long-distance relationship with my husband. I knew I needed meditation, relaxation, chamomile tea, and space just to be out in nature, but I was prioritizing everything (and everyone) else first. But when I fell apart and ended up in bed for more than two weeks, there was no "me" to hold it all together. I learned a lot from this. I learned that I could lean on other people, that delegating is the best thing ever, and that having a baked potato, crackers, and sliced cucumbers for dinner every now and then wouldn't kill my kid. But living the way I had been would kill me. So I learned to ask for help, to schedule in rest days and self-care time as if it were an important meeting, and lean on the ones who love me. This has saved my life and given me a much healthier relationship with my son and my business. The lesson here, I think, is to not fall apart before you make the changes. Start listening now, asking for help now, start scheduling in that "me" time, and gather support from your community and family. People are more willing to help then you think.

MOTHERING FROM THE HEART

Children are often punished for being human. They get cranky, they have bad days, they whine, they don't want to eat certain things, they make a mess, they don't want to go to school . . . just like us. We expect our children to behave and listen, but do we hold ourselves to the same standards? We snap at our children so quickly when they seem out of line or do something to embarrass us, but they are simply being children, being human. They are not meaning to hurt us, never vindictive or out to hurt anyone, children are just trying to get their needs met in whatever way they can. Sometimes that shows as acting out if they feel they can't get your attention any other way.

Recently we had a friend over for dinner. We were sitting at the table and my son, Henry, wanted to move chairs to sit next to his grandma. He walked across the top of the table. Both my husband and I felt embarrassed and quickly said, "absolutely not!" and basically publicly shamed him without even realizing what we were doing. He got to his seat and hung his head out of embarrassment. He didn't mean to do anything "bad," he just thought that was the quickest way to his seat. I quickly realized what I had done and went over to him to rewind. I said, "Honey, I know how important it is to you to sit next to Mimi, and I know how fun it is for you to walk and sit on the table, and I understand, and mommy would like to ask that you use the floor when we're eating." He heard me, hugged me, and hasn't done it since. I'm not saying a child shouldn't have boundaries here, but I leaned in and treated him like a person and not a "bad dog." He felt seen and like I respected him. It brought us closer and built respect, versus separating us and creating unhealthy shame. From that moment on, I've been handling situations in this way. Getting down on his level, acknowledging him, trying to see it from his angle, and then simply asking him for what I need or would like from him. When a child is treated with respect and seen as an equal human being, they feel it and they lean in, too.

TANTRUMS

Let me start this off by saying I have experienced a plethora of tantrums with Henry. Not just crying, but him hitting, pinching, punching, grabbing fistfuls of my hair, yelling at me, and letting me know how much he hates me. It's not easy. I know firsthand how triggering tantrums can be for a parent. I tried many different approaches and what I share below is what ultimately helped me heal some undercurrent wounds from my own childhood and allowed Henry to really feel what he needed to feel, then move on. Tantrums are more rare at our house now, but when they happen I feel very capable of handling him with love and compassion.

I believe tantrums are a beautiful opportunity to practice leaning in and getting closer to your child. If they are kicking and hitting you, it's okay to stay back. Something you can say so they know you are really caring is, "Mommy sees you need some space, I'll be right over here loving you. When you're ready to be close I'll be nearby." Then just sit a little bit away from your child and let them get the energy out. Sometimes a good kick and scream is what they need. Let them have it, but not on you. How good would it feel if we could do that and know someone was nearby loving us through it? You can also say small soothing words such as, "I'm here," "it's okay to have big feelings," or just a simple "mhmm." When they feel your true presence this will allow them to really let out what they need to and then move on. Often after a big tantrum, children will often go right into sweet playing and a very calm mood. Watch this and see what you notice with your child.

NOTE: If you have other children and it's disruptive, it's okay to bring your upset child into a room where you can be together while he goes through it. Watch your triggers. It's easy to get very angry when you feel your child's anger; pause for a little bit if you need to and remember you child is not meaning to be "bad"

they are just trying to let out something that is stuck.

The thing with tantrums is that they are usually the result of pent-up emotions a child didn't get the chance to release. By truly being with your child and not withdrawing love, they can feel that letting emotions out is a safe thing. By letting them have these full-on fits now, you will be helping them to connect deeper with themselves as they come into the teen years. When you are not forced to hold in emotions, you're less likely to try to soothe discomforts with food, alcohol, and drugs. Trust that there is nothing wrong with your child or you, it's just part of it, every child has tantrums and the way the parent handles them can either bring you closer or pull you further apart.

SHARING

This is often a big one for parents (myself included) because they feel it's a reflection of their personal character if their child doesn't share. It's not! Little ones usually aren't ready to share until around five years old. Young children need to feel a sense of "mine" and they need to feel you protect that. Don't worry, this won't last forever. What I've seen work so well with my child and many other little ones in my mother's kindergarten is letting your little one know that some friends are coming over and give her the opportunity to put away any toy she doesn't want to share. Let her leave out the ones that she does feel okay sharing. If you're in a situation, say at the park, and another child wants to play with your child's toy, don't make your little one give it up! You can simply say, "this is Jamie's toy, she's not quite ready to share it"—that's all! Forcing sharing before your child authentically feels the pull to share can be really confusing. They need to feel that you're on their side. They will come around to sharing—children are very giving by nature. Just let it come at its own speed.

I've found myself in several uncomfortable moments with sharing. I didn't follow my own advice at first because it felt socially wrong somehow, but the more I tuned into Henry and decided to go with what felt internally right, the easier sharing became. Henry felt that I was on his side, and I never forced him to share things that were dear to him. Now at almost six he is very happy to share and can clearly and kindly communicate when he doesn't feel comfortable sharing.

ONE-ON-ONE TIME

Children thrive when they get a little bit of our undivided attention each day. Even if it's just five minutes, giving your child that time can be an incredibly bonding and freeing act. By connecting with them one-on-one and just being with them to do whatever it is they please (within healthy limits, of course), you help them feel seen and loved. We call it "special time" at our house, and when we do it, our lives are easy! Especially if both my husband and I have busy days and we have to work a lot, we give Henry ten minutes of undivided time from each of us (separately), and the response is incredible. Henry will typically feel fed by that time with us and then be very happy to play independently while we take care of our adult needs. We always set a timer so he knows when it's over. He's come to depend on it and ask for it when he feels he needs to be really connected with one-on-one.

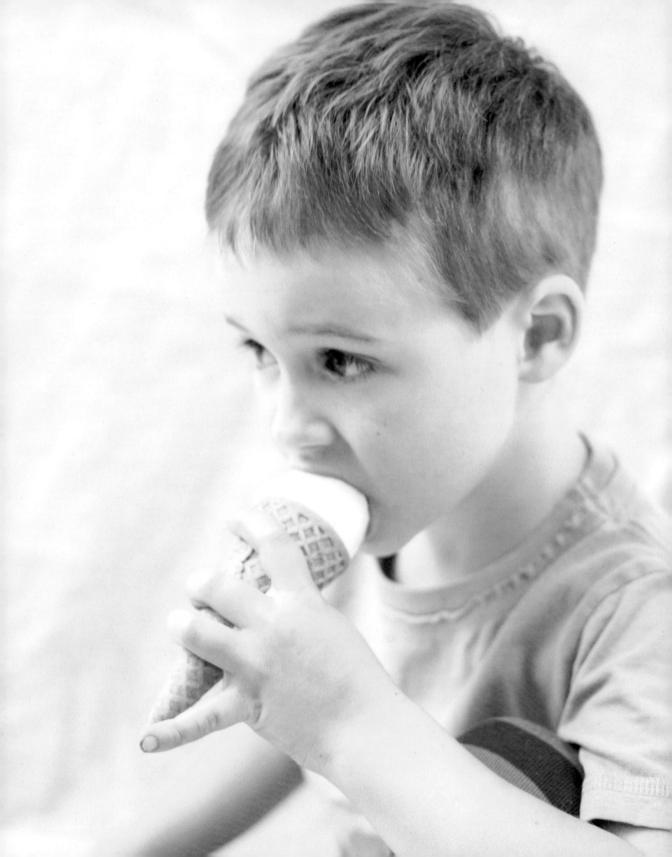

RHYTHM

Having a rhythm in the home can be such a blessing for both you and your child. It helps the family know what to expect. Having something solid to rely on really helps everyone relax. I post my rhythm on the refrigerator so that my husband and other caretakers are aware of the form we are trying to hold. It's really simple and can look however you want it to.

An example would be:

MORNING
Brush teeth and floss
Get dressed
Read two short story books together
Eat breakfast
Playtime

SCHOOL
9:00 a.m.–4:00 p.m.

AFTERNOON AND EVENING
Afternoon snack and library
Dinnertime
After-dinner walk
Story and nighttime routine
Prayer or family meditation

FAVORITE PARENTING BOOKS

The Aware Baby by Aletha J. Solter, PhD
Hold on to Your Kids by Gordon Neufeld, PhD and Gabor Maté, MD
Listen by Patty Wipfler and Tosha Schore
Rest, Play, Grow by Deborah MacNamara PhD
Tears and Tantrums by Aletha J. Solter, PhD
You are Your Child's First Teacher by Rahima Baldwin Dancy

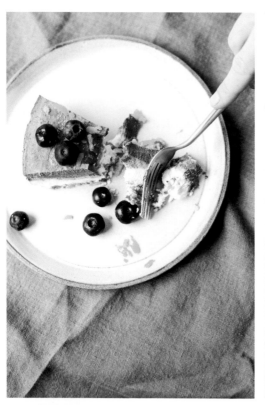

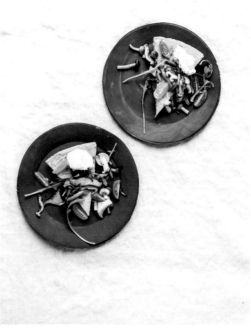

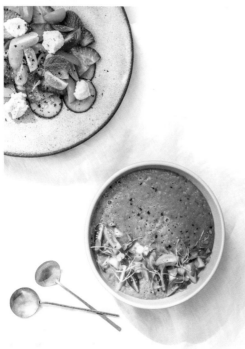

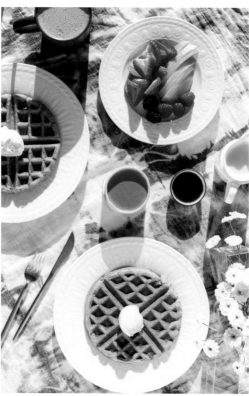

ON FOOD

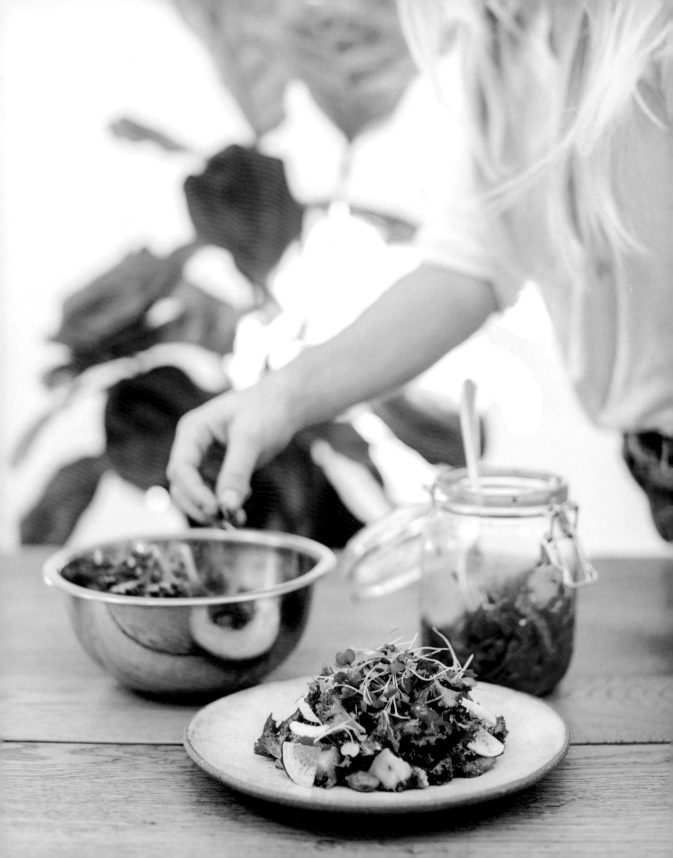

CONSCIOUS EATING

Caring for yourself in body, mind, and spirit is a full-time job. It takes dedication and awareness. It takes management and self-assessment. If you let one part of your self-care slip, it will affect the others. It's a holy trinity. When this triad is holistically tended to, your most authentic self shines though and creates an irresistible radiance. This part of the book focuses on physical nourishment.

Food has the ability to help open portals or to lock them shut. When you feed your body high-vibrational foods from the earth that radiate life, guess what, like becomes like. "You are what you eat" is an old saying but it's true. The food you eat literally becomes you! I've created these recipes to help you get on a path of soul nourishment. These are not just random recipes. They have intentions behind them, they have love in them, they have wisdom and important information in them, but it requires you to be in an aware and awake state while preparing them. I believe that food holds energy, I believe your emotional state affects your food (and your digestion), and I also support a short mediation or prayer of sorts before preparing these delicious meals. Give thanks, open up, ask for what you want, and channel it. I like to call these foods and practices conscious eating. It really is about so much more than just the food.

IN MY KITCHEN

The kitchen is my "inflow spot." I get in there and I go. It's expressive, it's therapeutic, it's sensual. It's a world of its own, and in my kitchen I'm the vessel through which magic travels. Food goes far beyond just the ingredients; the intention, the feeling behind it, the vibrations. . . . I consider myself a witch doctor of sorts, making meals that heal the heart and tap me back in, setting intentions and creating magic with what I make and serve. It's a sacred practice for me, not just a task to get done. It has deep meaning and is filled with more than meets the eye. Everyone always asks what the secret ingredient is. Here is a hint—it's not food based, it's not tangible. It's very much an energy and a vibration that can't be touched or even seen. The secret ingredient of everything powerful and amazing is always source energy that is flowing from within.

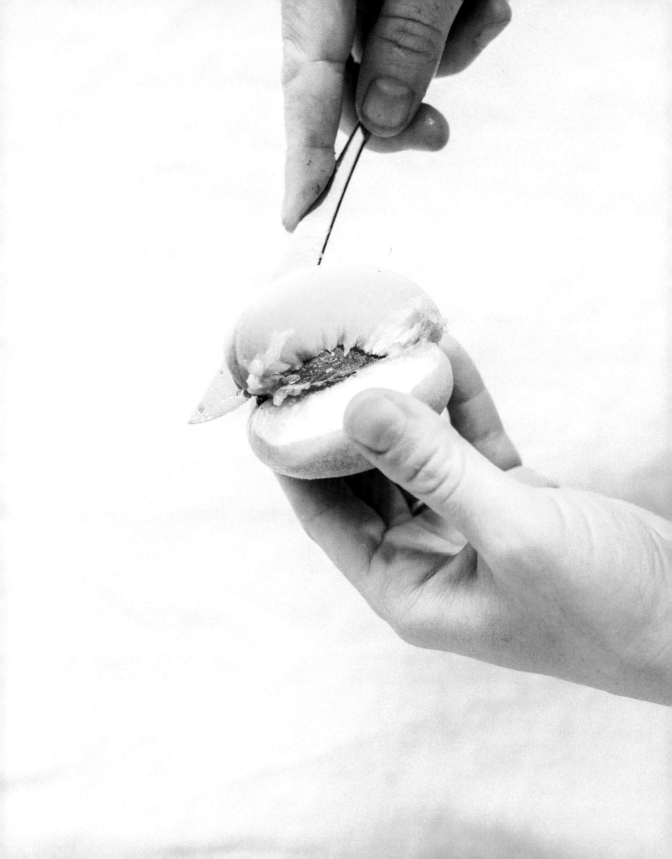

In my kitchen, you'll find an abundance of raw foods, fresh farmers' market fruits, vegetables, herbs, seeds, pasture-raised organic eggs, homemade bone broths, and once in a while some wild fish when in season. You also hear a sensual (not necessarily sexy, just really sense-oriented) playlist. I pull inspiration from many different cultures and food ethos. Working with healthy sprouted grains, seaweeds, broths, spices, fresh produce, and sometimes local organic pasture-raised animal products. I don't personally follow any diet type, I consider myself "flexitarian." I love to eat for pleasure and art—if I'm served a meal by gracious hosts, I eat it, I'm grateful, and I give thanks for the community and love that went into preparing the food. My day-to-day eating is grounded in plants. They make me feel radiant and have never failed me when it comes to healing myself. Food is medicine; it's a portal if you allow it to be. The intentions and methods of preparation have so much to do with our full-bodied wellness.

This book is grounded in plant-based wisdom, and I share some recipes that include eggs and also bone broths, but I support you to eat in a way that makes you feel amazing! If eating a little wild-caught fish or grass-fed beef makes you feel great, then enjoy it fully. And on the contrary, if animal products don't match where your heart and body are at, don't do it! I eat what gives me pleasure and lasting health, knowing that pleasure supports my lasting health! So, if that chocolate cakes gives you lasting pleasure, then let yourself have that opportunity from time to time. For me, it's about eating clean and as close to the earth as possible (most of the time), blessing the food that nourishes me and being conscious while I'm dining. Living this way makes room for that pleasure food here and there with no huge harm to your body. I use my intuition and choose foods that feel great to me. I also am really aware of my full self, my full body. Making choices from a place of love and intention versus pain and conditioning has been a huge part of my personal inner work.

Everyone will have an opinion when it comes to food. What I support you to do is feel into what makes you feel your best—no one knows you like you! My baseline guidance is to choose organic locally sourced foods whenever possible and if you're consuming animal products, choose only local organic and pasture raised. This is not only healthier for you but also for our planet. Eating and shopping local is a wonderful way to support your local farms and keep the dollars in your community.

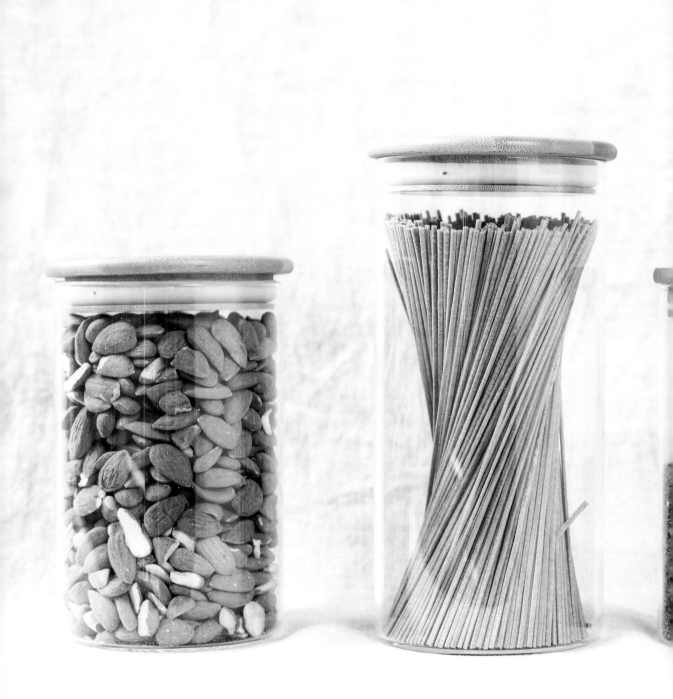

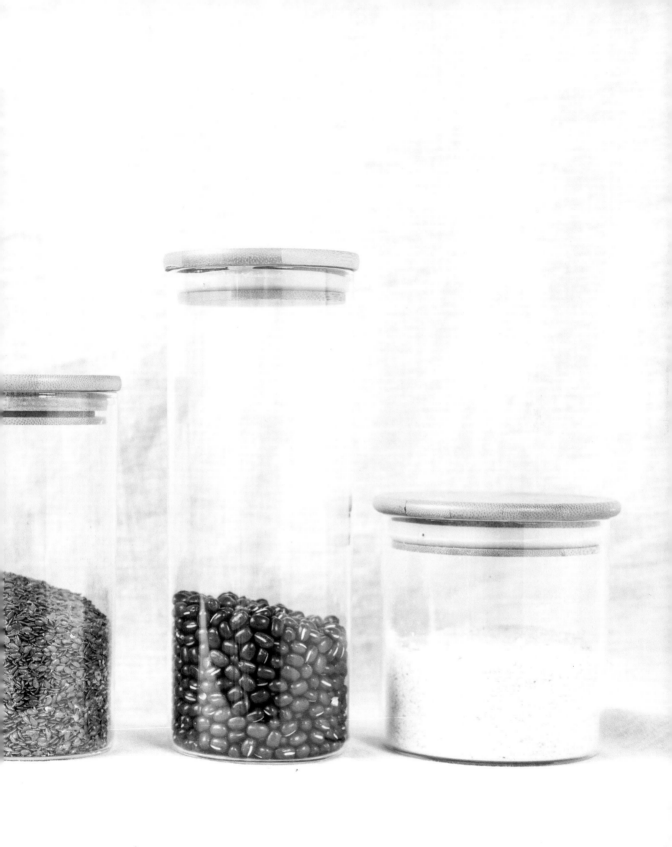

PANTRY

A simple list of foods that I love to have on hand for easy-to-make meals.

GRAINS, NUTS, SEEDS + LEGUMES

Remember to always soak grains, seeds, and legumes—see my soaking chart on page 280.

Adzuki beans

Almonds

Amaranth

Black beans

Buckwheat

Buckwheat noodles

Cashews

Gluten-free oats

Hazelnuts

Lentils

Macadamia nuts

Pepitas or pumpkin seeds

Quinoa

Sesame seeds

Sprouted brown rice

Sunflower seeds

Walnuts

OILS + FLOURS + MISC

Almond flour

Apple cider vinegar

Brown rice flour

Citrus

Coconut flour

Cold-pressed macadamia nut oil

Cold-pressed organic coconut oil

Extra-virgin olive oil

Grass-fed cultured raw butter

Grass-fed ghee

Good-quality protein powder

Salt*

Stone-ground almond butter

Stone-ground coconut butter

*Great salt is key to great food and flavoring, and good-quality salt can change the flavor of your meal. Salt is a wonderful flavor enhancer and will really bring out the sweet, spice, and herbal flavors. Choosing the right salt is important for your health and your food's flavor. I love Celtic salt, Maldon Sea Salt, and pink salt. I use all three of these throughout the recipes in this book.

FAVORITE SPICES + FLAVORS

Almond extract

Black pepper

Cardamom

Chipotle

Cinnamon

Coriander

Cumin

Curry spice

Nutmeg

Orange oil

Vanilla beans

HEALTHY SWEETENERS

Brown rice syrup

Dates

Fruit juice

Maple syrup

Monk fruit

Raw honey

Stevia (must be pure stevia, no natural flavors; I love Omica)

FAVORITE SUPERFOODS

Bee pollen

Chia

Chlorella

Coconut oil

Collagen

Colostrum

Flax

Goji berries

Maca

Matcha

Raw cacao

Spirulina

Wheatgrass, powdered or fresh

HERBS + MUSHROOMS

Astragalus

Chaga

Chamomile

Cordyceps

Dandelion root

He shou wu

Lion's mane

Mint

Nettles

Rhodiola

Reishi

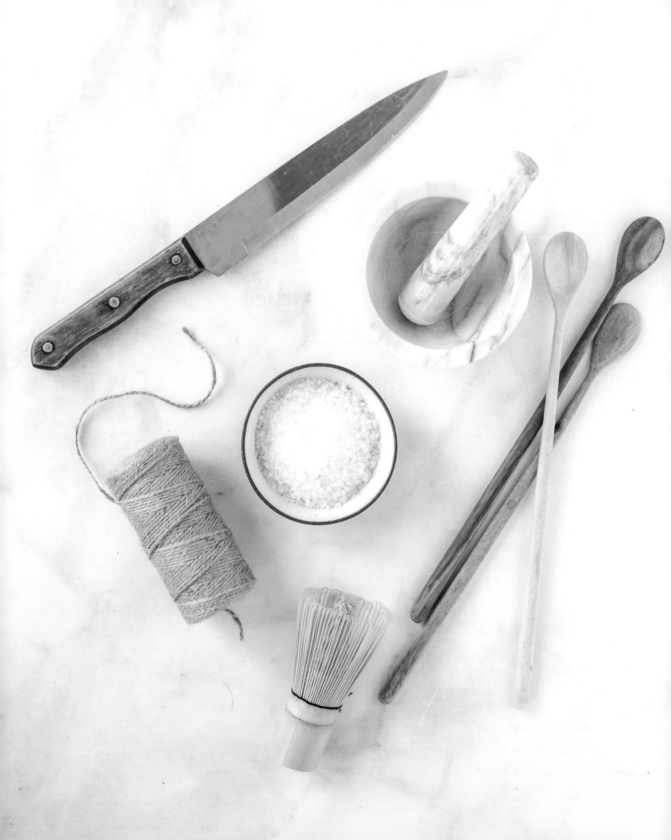

KITCHEN TOOLS

A list of kitchen tools that make all these recipes and many others a breeze. You don't need all of these to make these recipes, but it always is nice to have a well-stocked kitchen that's ready for anything.

CAST-IRON SKILLET

Perfect for making sauces, braising greens, sautéing vegetables, and making pancakes. I love cast iron because it's clean. I steer clear of all Teflon and aluminum cookware, opting for toxin-free metals such as cast iron and stainless steel. I also use clay and stone cookware.

TONGS

Great for plating and making things lovely! Always good to have for hot foods and salads.

NUT MILK BAGS

I have a love affair with nut and seed milks. You'll find a lot of recipes in this book that require nut milk bags. You find can find them online (Amazon has a ton!) or just use cheesecloth if you are eager to get started!

WHISK

A good whisk is important for baked goods, pancakes, sauces, and smoothing bumps out of flours and tonic herbs.

OFFSET SPATULA

Some of the raw food items in this book will require an offset spatula for spreading. Also great for icing cakes.

WOODEN SPOON

I think of these like an heirloom. Something a mother passes down to her daughter and so on. Great for stirring your sauces and stews.

BENCH SCRAPER

One of my must have kitchen tools, I mainly use it for scoring raw foods and for cleaning off my cutting board.

Y-SHAPED PEELER

You'll need this for so many things: salads, fruits, veggie noodles—it's a great and relatively cheap investment.

KNIFE SET

I feel that having a good knife set is paramount when setting up a kitchen. I use Shen knives and really take care of them. This is an investment but one that will pay off.

COOKIE SHEET

A good stainless steel or ceramic baking sheet will come in handy for roasting veggies, making sweet potato fries, and of course, cookies!

SPRINGFORM PAN

Many of the raw food and baked treats require a springform pan. They make it really easy to remove the dessert from with no mess. It's hard to find springform pan that are not made of Teflon or aluminum. I typically use these primarily for raw treats and since nothing is heated in them, they are safe.

FOOD PROCESSOR

Second only to Vitamix in my kitchen, I use my food processor for so many things.

VITAMIX

My number one kitchen tool, this will change your life if it hasn't already. From smoothies to sauces, blended soups to cookie batter, this is hands down the best kitchen investment you'll ever make.

MICROPLANE

A small grater that can give you quick and easy citrus zest (or any zest).

SOUP POT

Having a great soup pot that won't burn on the bottom is paramount! I like stainless steel or ceramic cook pots.

GLASS JARS FOR INGREDIENTS

This is how I organize my pantry, having everything visible helps me know what and how much I have on hand of each ingredient.

PLASTIC SQUEEZE BOTTLES

Important for plating and topping. Great place for storing dressings as well.

METAL SPATULA

Metal spatulas are great for scoring and for really getting clean lines with food. I use them for all French toasts, pancakes, and baking.

GOOD KITCHEN SCISSORS

Always important, they come in handy for more things then you would ever think. We even cut our pizza with them!

SPIRALIZER

Make your own vegetable noodles! This is great for raw, vegan, and Paleo diet types. You can eat the noodles raw or cook them. A great healthy alternative.

DEHYDRATOR

This is not needed, you can use an oven, but it's pretty awesome to get one for raw foods. You can find them on Amazon for around $100 to $200. A fun and worthwhile kitchen investment.

AEROLATTE

This is such a fun tool for foamy lattes and tonics.

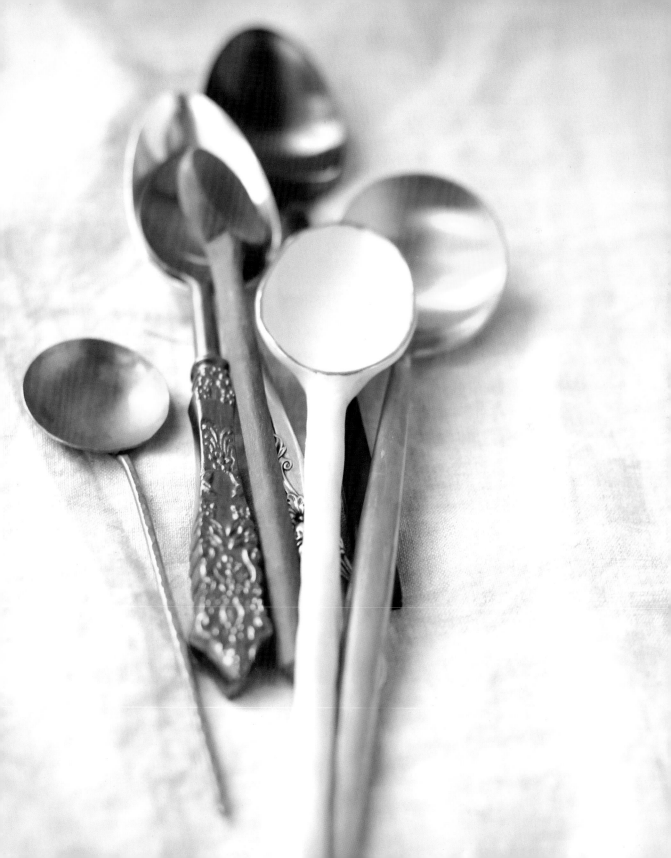

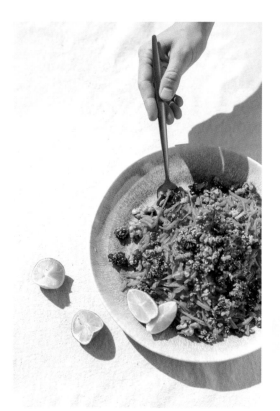
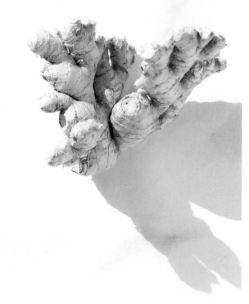
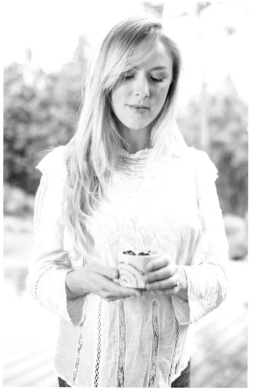
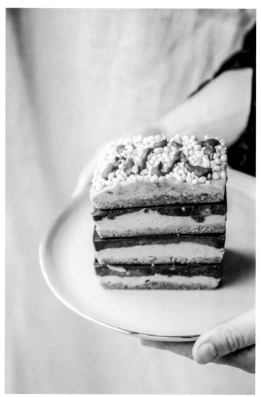

THE RECIPES

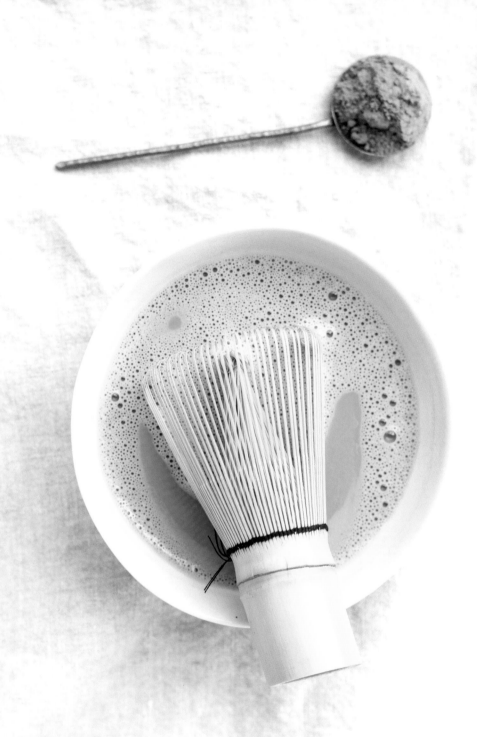

Matcha Latte, page 89

TONICS, COFFEES + TEAS

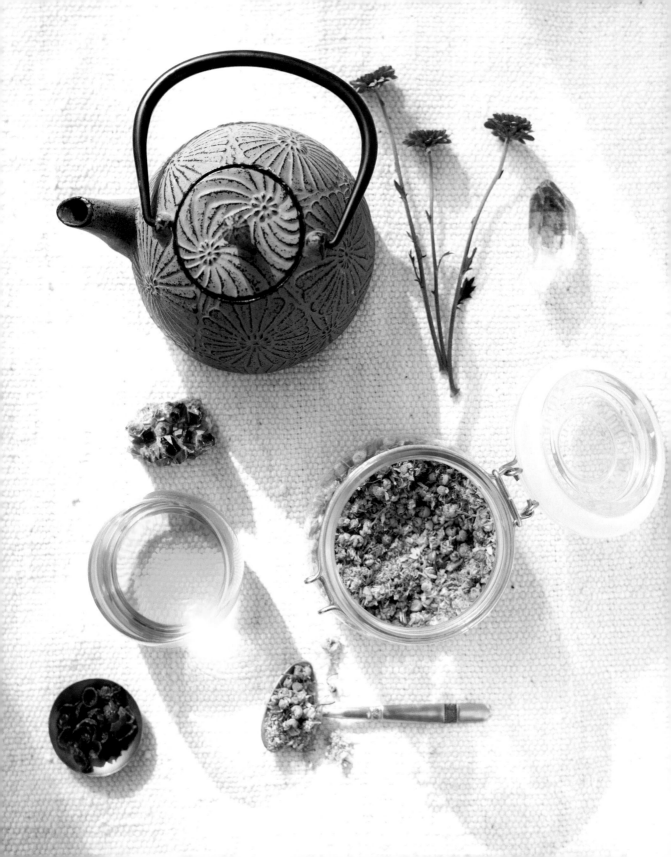

SUN + MOON TEA

This is tea that is made by exposing the herbs to the energy of the sun or moon. There is so much that goes unseen energetically speaking and I love the idea that when we put our foods (and bodies) in front of the sun or moon they get charged with specific energies that enhance our life force. This tea-making method calls on some principles of biodynamic farming. I love the concept and I love the tea! Give it a try. It's very fun to do with children; they seem to understand the connection naturally. These herbs can be found online, I love www.moun tainroseherbs.com

Makes 8 Servings

7 cups water
¼ cup peppermint leaves
¼ cup chamomile leaves
¼ cup lemon balm
1 cup red clover flowers
1 cup orange peel

Combine the water and herbs in a large 8-cup glass container.

Let sit overnight or through the day for two nights or days.

Use a large strainer to remove herbs.

Store in the refrigerator for up to 7 days.

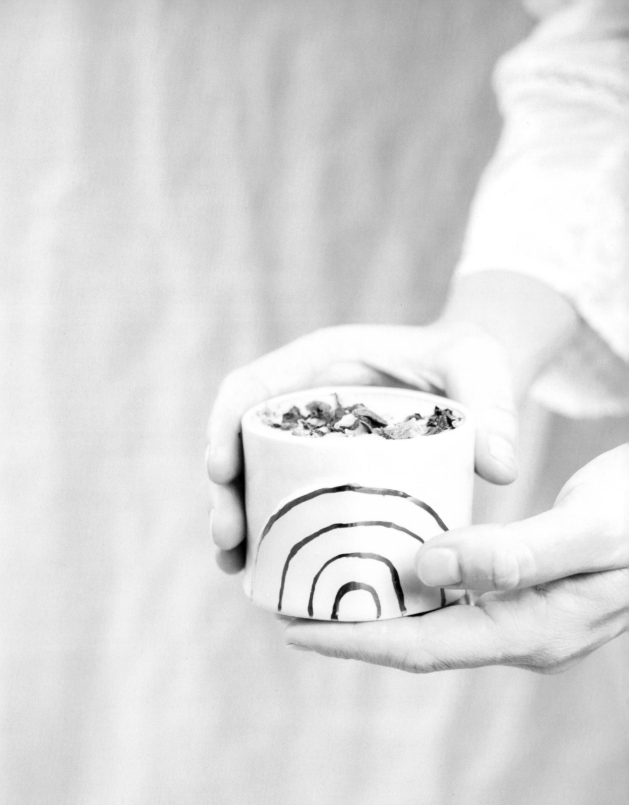

BEAUTY TONIC LATTE

Morning tonics are a great way to get a ton of nutrition into one small cup. This is a beauty tonic but also has a good amount of protein and energizing superfoods. Collagen is one of the best ways to support your gut, your skin, your hair, and your ligaments. There are vegan versions as well as animal-based. I love Moon Juice for a plant-based option. If you are opting for a non vegan option, Bulletproof has a very clean version. Pearl Powder, schisandra, and cacao are all beauty-promoting superfoods that are high in minerals, antioxidants, and skin protecting properties.

Makes 1 Serving

1½ cups macadamia nut milk
   (page 102)
2 tablespoons raw cacao powder
1 tablespoon collagen protein
   (Moon Juice has a great vegan
   version called Beauty Shroom)
½ teaspoon pearl powder
½ teaspoon schisandra
2 teaspoons maple syrup or
   3 drops Omica stevia
1 tablespoon stone-ground
   almond or stone-ground
   coconut butter
⅛ teaspoon pink salt
Dried roses for topping (optional)

If making a hot version, heat your milk to 175° F. If making a cold version, skip to step 2.

Add all ingredients (except roses) into a blender and blend on high for 1 minute.

Pour into your favorite mug, decorate with dried roses if desired, and enjoy!

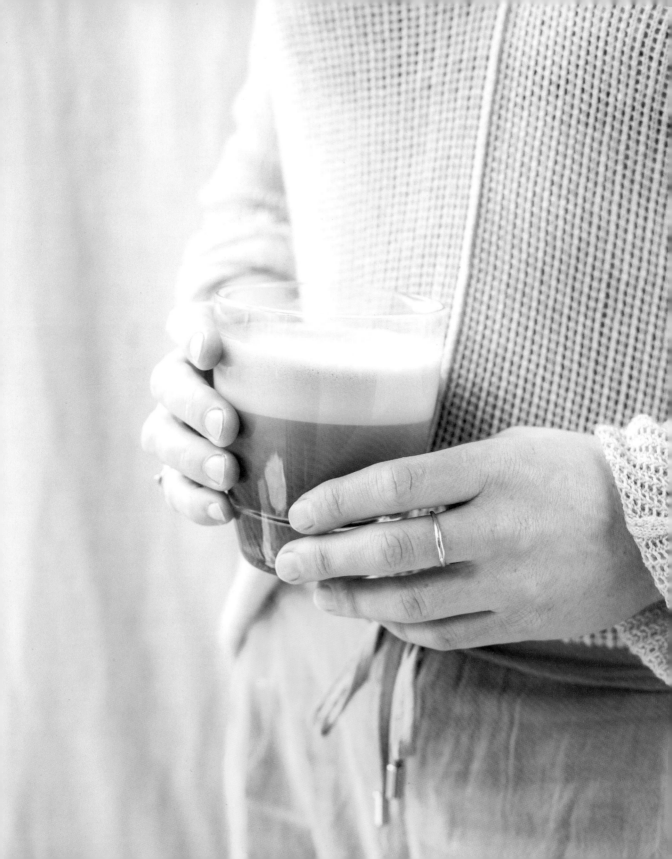

HAUTE CHOCOLATE

Super sexy stuff. Luxurious and self-indulgent just as it should be. Enjoy!

Makes 2 Serving

1½ cups macadamia nut milk (page 102)
2 tablespoons stone-ground almond butter
½ teaspoon cordyceps
1 tablespoon tocotrienols (fat-soluble vitamin E)
2 tablespoons raw cacao powder
⅛ teaspoon pink salt

If making a hot version, heat your milk to 175°F. If making a cold version, skip to next step.

Add all ingredients into a blender and blend on high for 1 minute.

Pour into your favorite mug and enjoy!

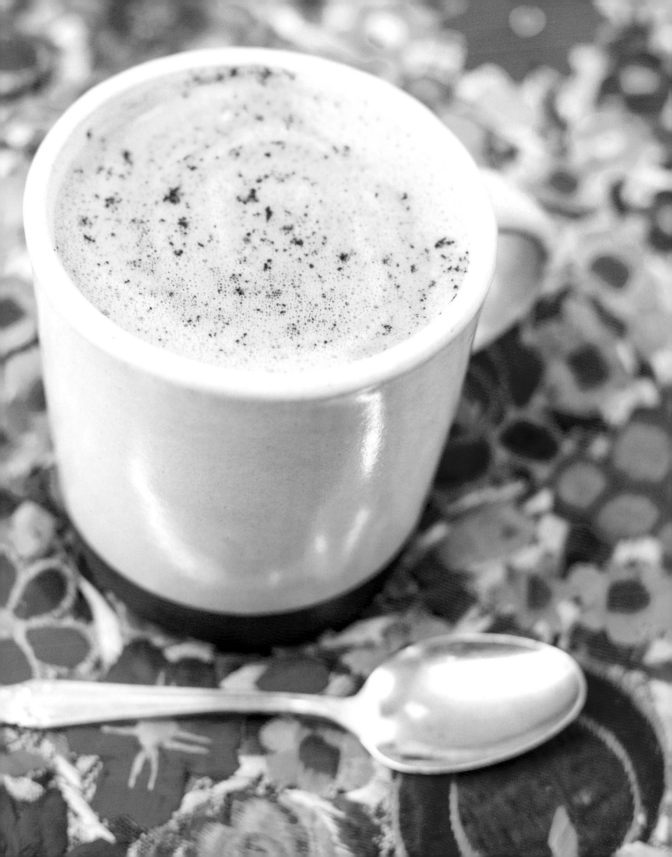

OAXACAN MOCHA

I love calling on Mexico for inspiration. I especially love Oaxaca. I still can see the vibrancy of that city in my mind's eye. When I first arrived I remember driving from the airport and even in the grayest areas of the city I felt life. I got to spend time in a small village that was incredibly off the grid. I was touched by how kind the people were. They took us in, fed us, and treated us as family. These were people who had hardly anything. The floors of the house were dirt, yet they gave us everything they had and with joy. It felt so real. So alive on a level that I rarely experience in the States. So I named this concoction Oaxacan, because the cacao and spices help to open the heart and awaken a sense of oneness.

Makes 1 Serving

1½ cups brewed organic fair-trade coffee (ideally locally roasted!)

2 tablespoons stone-ground almond butter

2 tablespoons raw cacao powder

¼ teaspoon cinnamon

⅛ teaspoon nutmeg

⅛ teaspoon anise seeds

⅛ teaspoon chili powder

⅛ teaspoon pink salt

2 teaspoons maple syrup or 4 drops Omica stevia

If making a hot version, use your brewed coffee. If making a cold version, use premade cold-brew coffee.

Add all ingredients into a blender and blend on high for 1 minute.

Pour into your favorite mug and enjoy!

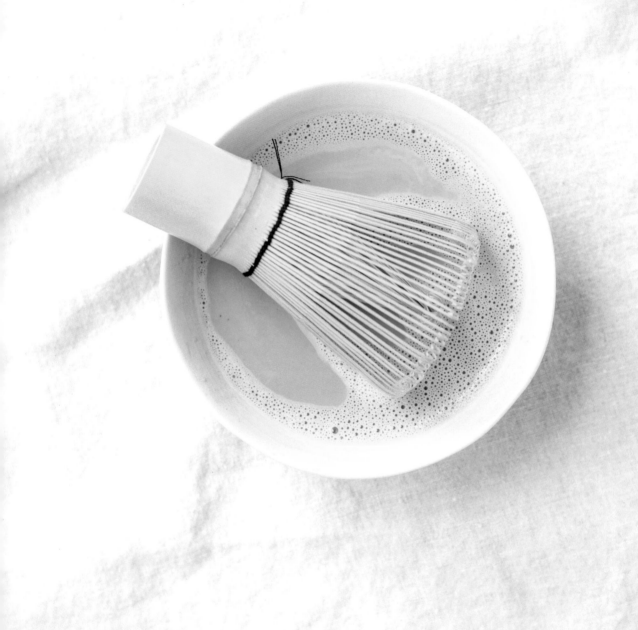

MATCHA LATTE

I have a long-term love affair with matcha. We even sell our own ceremonial-grade matcha called Gaia Matcha at Local Juicery (www.localjuicery.com). I'm enamored with it. I love its feminine feel and its soft and subtle uplifting qualities. Matcha is filled with powerful antioxidants including the amazing EGCg (thought to boost your metabolism and slow or halt the growth of cancer), it boosts the immune system, contains skin-loving chlorophyll, and just plain tastes amazing. Matcha can really be added to any smoothie or tonic, but I love to taste the flavor. Enjoy this matcha latte hot or cold! I suggest buying matcha that is only sourced from Japan, as it tests the cleanest for heavy metals and is made authentically.

Makes 1 Serving

1½ cups almond milk (page 101)
1 teaspoon ceremonial-grade
  matcha green tea powder
2 teaspoons maple syrup or
  3 drops Omica stevia
1 tablespoon stone-ground
  almond or stone-ground
  coconut butter
Pinch pink salt

If making a hot version, heat your milk to 170°F. If cold, move to next step.

Add all ingredients into a blender and blend on high for 1 minute.

Pour into your favorite mug and enjoy!

NOTE: You can also use a matcha whisk for the recipe—you would blend the almond milk, maple syrup, nut butter, and salt in the blender and then whisk in a bowl with a matcha whisk as pictured.

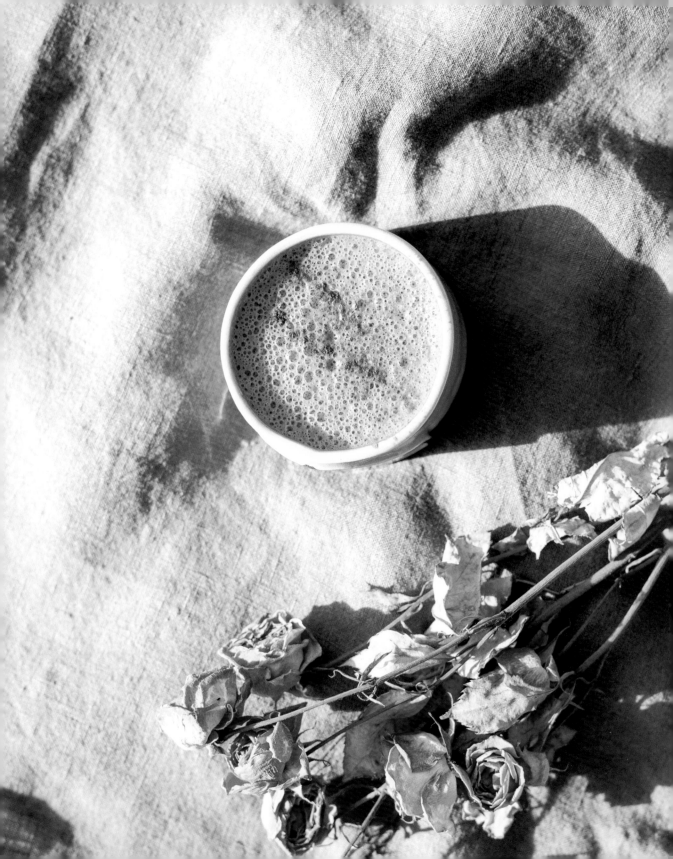

PREGNANCY TONIC

Cutting caffeine is often hard for new mamas-to-be, especially if they are working mamas or already have children. It's hard to cut something that we often lean on so heavily, but it's also really important to omit it. Using this alternative tea tonic will help soothe the body and give you energy in the morning but without the caffeine. I love adding ghee or grass-fed butter to this for good fats, but if you're a vegan feel free to use coconut butter or oil!

Makes 1 Serving

1½ cups brewed raspberry-leaf tea (hot or cold based on preference)

1 tablespoon grass-fed butter, ghee, or coconut butter

1 tablespoon plant or collagen protein

½ teaspoon turmeric powder (optional)

½ teaspoon cinnamon

⅛ teaspoon cardamom

Maple syrup to taste

¼ teaspoon pearl powder

⅛ teaspoon pink salt

Add all ingredients into a blender and blend on high for 1 minute.

Pour into your favorite mug and enjoy!

NOTE: There are a couple different schools of thought when it comes to turmeric and pregnancy—some love it, some don't. I've used it in both my pregnancies and enjoyed the benefits. Please do your own research and always consult with your natural health care provider before using any herb or medicinal roots.

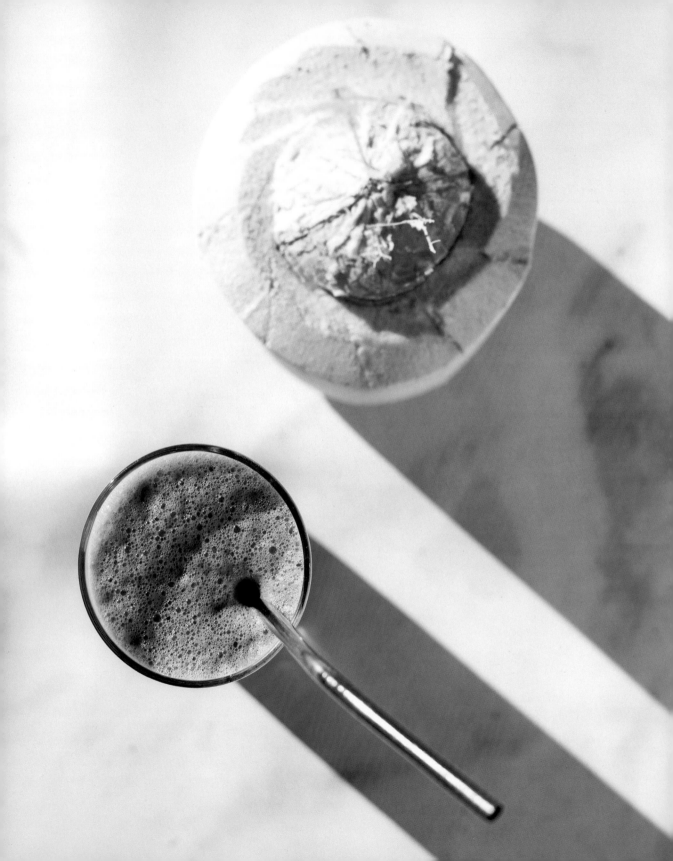

COCONUT MATCHA

Simply perfect for a hot summer day. All you need are two ingredients: young coconut and matcha powder.

Makes 1 Serving

---

1 young coconut, flesh removed
1½ teaspoons matcha powder

Combine coconut water and matcha in a blender and blend on high for 15 to 20 seconds.

Pour in a clear glass so you can admire the color and enjoy! Great with ice cubes!

MOTHER'S HELPER

I've struggled (like 99.9 percent of parents) with getting enough greens and healthy fats into my boy. He's five years old (upon writing this) and full of vim and vigor, but he'll get so into whatever he's doing that at times he'll forget to eat unless I force it on him. I came up with this recipe to get healthy fats and greens in him early in the morning that would keep him full for the entire morning. It's turned into a household favorite! The MCT oil is a great healthy medium-chain fatty acid that supports brain function. I use Bulletproof brand because it is sourced from 100 percent coconut versus palm oil.

Makes 1 Serving

1½ cups almond milk or favorite nut milk (page 101)
2 teaspoons raw cacao powder (I go light when I'm making for kiddos)
2 teaspoons barley grass powder, or favorite superfood green powder
2 tablespoons stone-ground almond butter
1 scoop favorite plant-based protein powder
½ teaspoon reishi mushroom powder
1 teaspoon MCT oil
5 drops Omica stevia
⅛ teaspoon pink salt

If making a hot version, heat the milk on the stove until it is warm to the touch. If making a cold version, skip to the next step.

Add all ingredients into a blender and blend on high for 1 minute.

Pour into your favorite mug and enjoy!

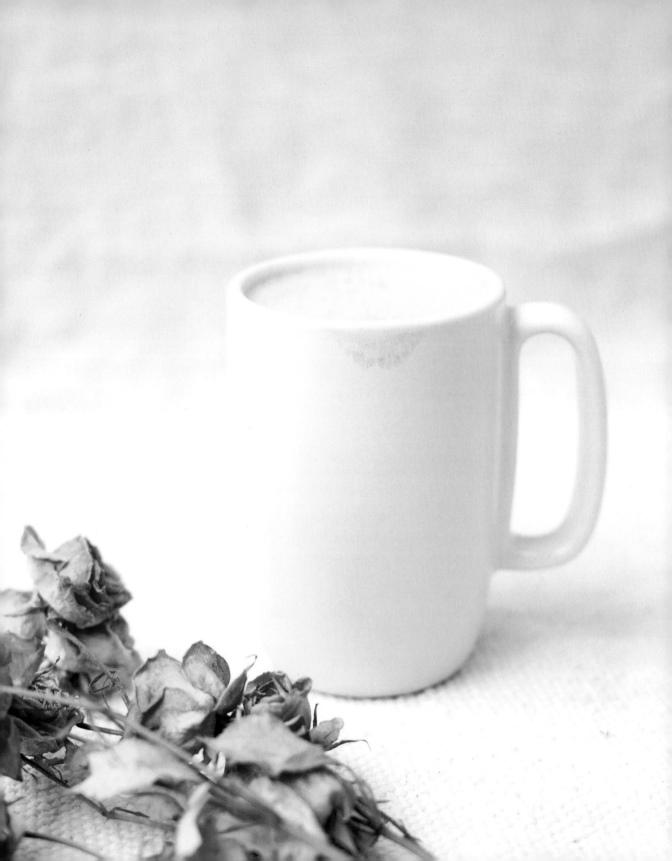

VITALITY COFFEE

The name says it all. If you're in need of a major energy boost, this is the one. It features medicinal mushrooms, cacao, and maca. You'll be blasting off!

Makes 1 Serving

1½ cups brewed organic fair-trade coffee (ideally locally roasted!)
2 tablespoons stone-ground almond butter
¼ teaspoon reishi mushroom powder
¼ teaspoon cordyceps mushroom powder
¼ teaspoon he shou wu root
1 teaspoon maca powder
2 teaspoons raw cacao powder
2 teaspoons maple syrup or 4 drops Omica stevia
Pinch of salt

If making a hot version, use your brewed coffee. If making a cold version, use premade cold-brew coffee.

Add all ingredients into a blender and blend on high for 1 minute.

Pour into your favorite mug and enjoy!

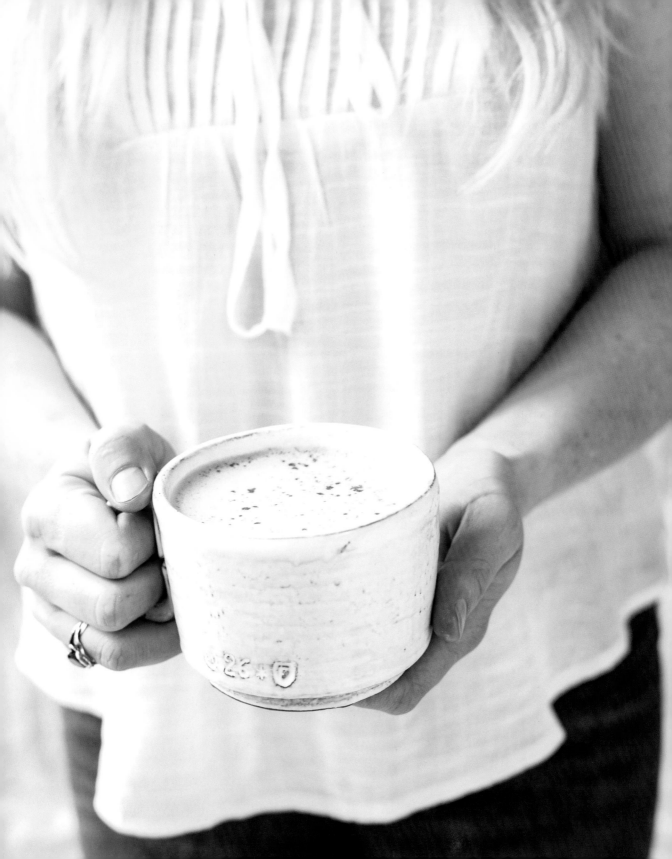

PRETTY PROTEIN TONIC

This is my on-the-go morning breakfast. The days when my kid won't get dressed and I can hardly get my face washed kind of breakfast. It's easy, full of protein, and can be made hot or cold depending on the season. I love it because the cacao helps me power through while the fats ground me and keep me full for a long time.

Makes 1 Serving

1½ cups nut milk of choice
2 tablespoons stone-ground almond butter
1 tablespoon maca
1 teaspoon coconut oil or grass-fed butter
1 tablespoon plant-based protein powder
3 tablespoons hemp seeds
teaspoon bee pollen
2 teaspoons maple syrup or 4 drops Omica stevia
Pinch of salt

If making a hot version, heat your milk to 175° F. If making a cold version, skip to step 2.

Add all ingredients into a blender and blend on high for 1 minute.

Pour into your favorite mug and enjoy!

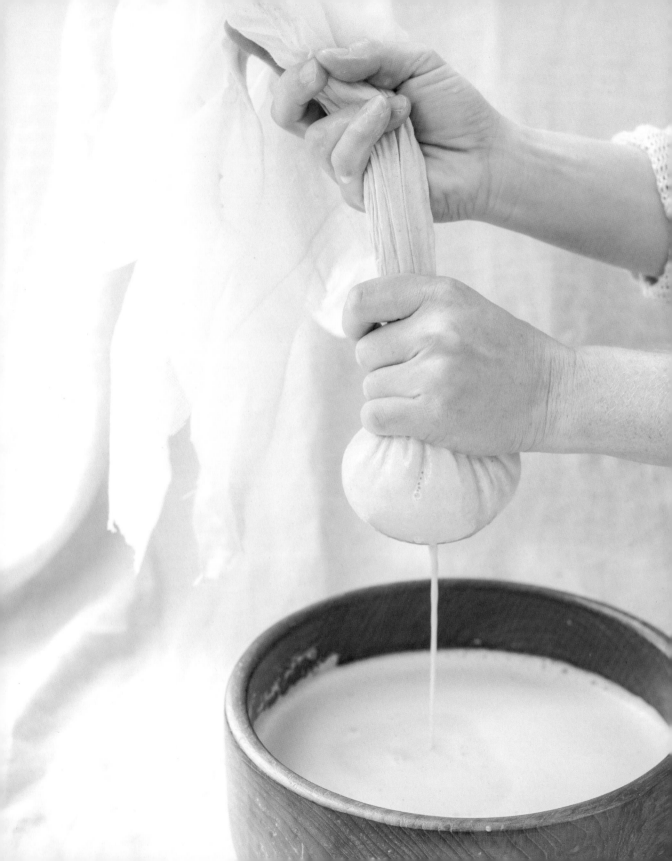

NUT MILKS

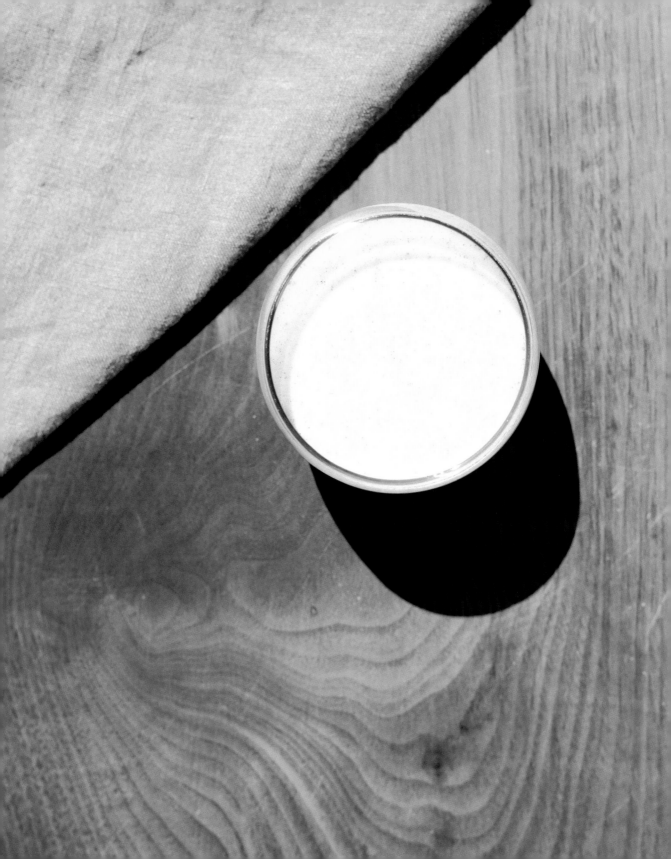

BASIC ALTERNATIVE MILK

This is a pretty standard ratio for nut and seed milks—you can use it across the board. But do reference the soaking chart for nuts and seeds on page 279 to make sure you're activating all the powerful nutrients from your food and avoiding nutrient blockers such as phytic acid. Store all nut and seed milks in the refrigerator after making. If you are soaking nuts or seeds, I always recommend soaking them in the refrigerator to keep them from spoiling too quickly.

Makes 4 Servings

1 cup soaked nuts, grains, or seeds
4 cups filtered water
3–4 dates, pitted
¼ teaspoon vanilla bean
½ teaspoon pink salt

Combine nuts, seeds, or grain of choice, water, dates, vanilla, and salt in a blender and blend on high until perfectly creamy.

Strain with a nut milk bag or cheesecloth.

Pour into a glass jar, seal, and keep in the refrigerator. Keeps for about 6 days.

1-MINUTE ALTERNATIVE MILK

The quick fix for when you need nut milk in a hurry. I use this 90 percent of the time! It's great for smoothies, lattes, tonics, and coffee creamer, and the best part is that it takes literally 1 minute to make.

Makes 2 Servings

2 cups water
½ cup nut or seed butter of choice
Maple syrup or favorite liquid sweetener of choice
¼ teaspoon pink salt

Combine water, nut or seed butter, sweetener, and salt in a blender and blend on high until perfectly creamy.

Pour into a glass jar, seal, and keep in the refrigerator. Keeps for about 6 days.

BRAZIL NUT MILK

Makes 4 servings

---

1 cup Brazil nuts, soaked
4 cups water
4–5 dates, pitted
¼ teaspoon salt

Combine Brazil nuts, water, dates, and salt in a blender and blend on high until perfectly creamy.

Strain with a nut milk bag or cheesecloth. Pour into a glass jar, seal, and keep in the refrigerator. Keeps for about 6 days.

MACADAMIA NUT MILK

Probably the most delicious milk of the bunch, but also the most pricey! I only make this once in a while. It's worth tasting and making when you feel like splurging.
Makes 4 Servings

---

1 cup macadamia nuts, soaked
4 cups water
4–5 dates, pitted
¼ teaspoon salt

Combine macadamia nuts, water, dates, and salt in a blender and blend on high until perfectly creamy.

Strain with a nut milk bag or cheesecloth. Pour into a glass jar, seal, and keep in the refrigerator. Keeps for about 6 days.

COCONUT MILK

I use young coconuts for my coconut milk, but you can use dried coconut as well. The benefits of young coconut are incredible, so hydrating, alkalizing, and full of natural electrolytes. Many Asian markets sell these coconuts for half the price of traditional grocery stores!
Makes 4 Servings

---

2 cups young coconut meat
4½ cups young coconut water
¼ teaspoon pink salt

Combine coconut meat, coconut water, and salt in a blender and blend on high until perfectly creamy. There is no need to strain this milk, but you can if you would like. I recommend using a metal strainer instead of a cloth for this recipe.

Pour into a glass jar, seal, and keep in the refrigerator. Keeps for about 6 days.

ROASTED HAZELNUT MILK

The best milk in the world. I don't know how else to describe it. It goes well with everything.

Makes 4 Servings

2 cups hazelnuts, roasted
4 cups water
4–5 dates, pitted
½ teaspoon salt

Preheat the oven to 350°F. Place hazelnuts on a baking sheet and bake for 15 minutes or until golden brown. Let the hazelnuts cool and then pour into a blender.

Add water, dates, and salt, and blend until smooth. Strain with a nut milk bag or cheesecloth. Pour into a glass jar, seal, and keep in the refrigerator. This milk will keep in the refrigerator for about 6 days.

ROASTED HAZELNUT CHOCOLATE MILK

A winner for everyone. Who can resist creamy chocolate milk? Not me! So I made this healthy version! It's especially amazing with the roasted hazelnut milk.

Makes 2 Cups

2 cups Roasted Hazelnut Milk
 (above)
3 tablespoons raw cacao powder
2 teaspoons maple syrup
¼ teaspoon pink salt

Combine hazelnut milk, cacao powder, maple syrup, and salt in a blender and blend on high until perfectly creamy.

Pour into a glass and enjoy!

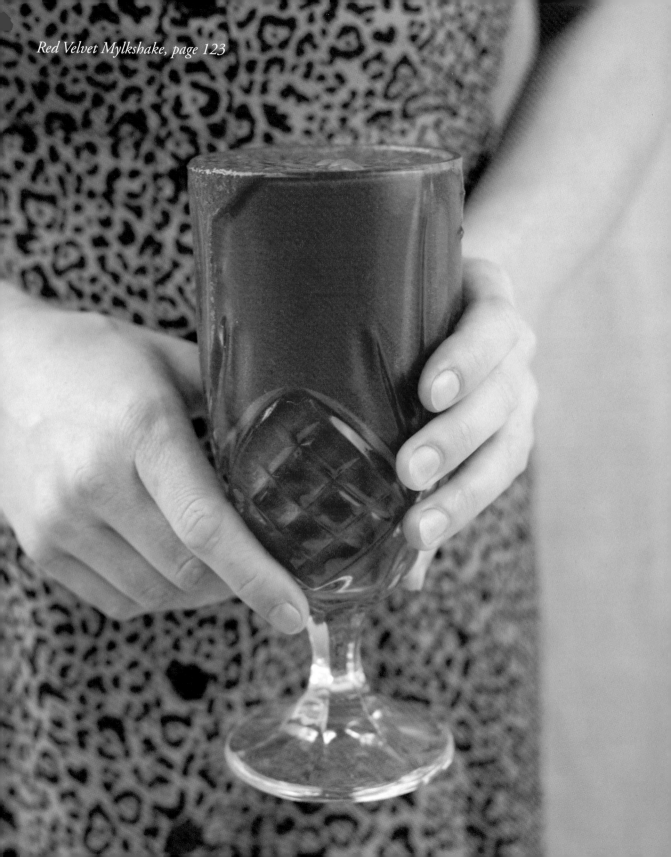

Red Velvet Mylkshake, page 123

SMOOTHIES + SHAKES

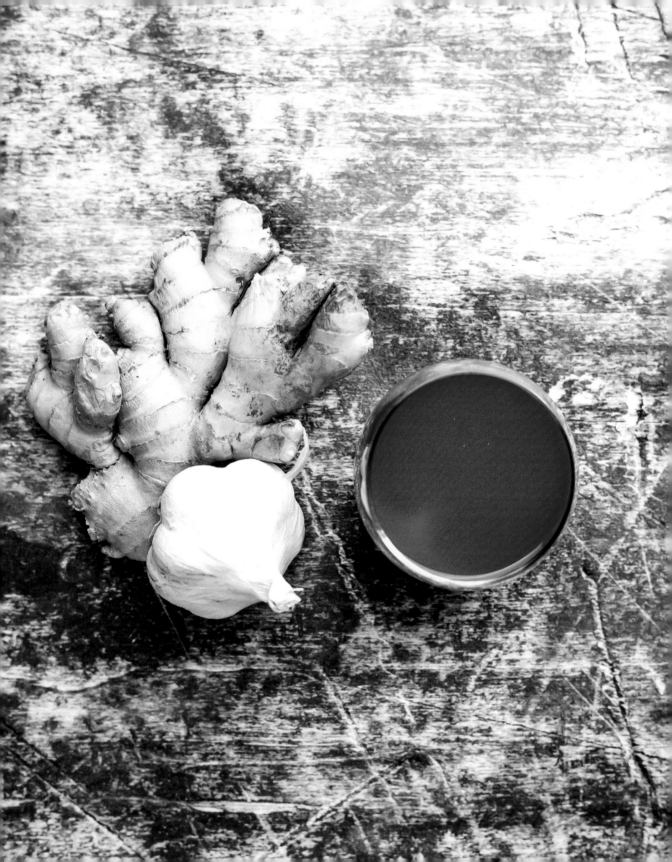

COLD KICKER

Forget flu shots, take this instead. It's loaded and will help knock out any sick bugs threatening your immune system. We have a version of this recipe at my shops, and around flu season I have clients who swear by it. They start taking it when the season starts and report back that the flu never gets them when they constantly drink this. The great thing about this recipe is all the citrus and spices act as a natural preservative. It will last 2 weeks or more in the refrigerator. I recommended tripling the recipe and making a big pitcher when you're feeling low.

Makes 4 Servings

---

1 cup orange juice (best if made fresh)
4 ounces beet juice (optional)
1 tablespoon minced ginger
1 tablespoon minced turmeric
1 teaspoon black peppercorns
1–2 garlic cloves
1 tablespoon apple cider vinegar
¼ teaspoon pink salt
⅛ teaspoon cayenne pepper

Combine all ingredients in your blender and blend on high for 30 seconds.

Run through a mesh strainer and discard pulp

Pour into your favorite shot glass and drink up.

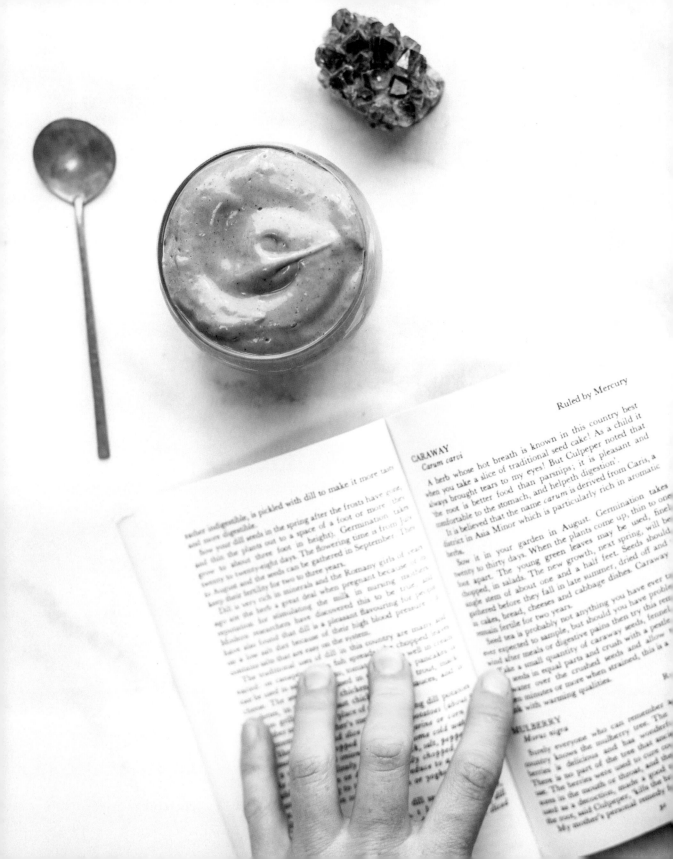

CARAWAY
Carum carvi

A herb whose hot breath is known in this country best when you take a slice of traditional seed cake! As a child it always brought tears to my eyes! But Culpeper noted that the root is better food than parsnips; it is pleasant and comfortable to the stomach, and helpeth digestion'.

It is believed that the name *carum* is derived from Caria, a district in Asia Minor which is particularly rich in aromatic herbs.

Sow it in your garden in August. Germination takes twenty to thirty days. When the plants come up, thin to one foot apart. The young green leaves may be used, finely chopped, in salads. The new growth, next spring, will be a single stem of about one and a half feet. Seeds should be gathered before they fall in late summer, dried off and ...

... in cakes, bread, cheeses and cabbage dishes. Caraway remain fertile for two years.

... seed tea is probably not anything you have ever tasted ... expected to sample, but should you have problems ... wind after meals or digestive pains then try this remedy ... Take a small quantity of caraway seeds, fennel ... seeds in equal parts and crush with a pestle ... water over the crushed seeds and allow ... minutes or more when strained, this is a ... with warming qualities.

MULBERRY
Morus nigra

Surely everyone who can remember ... country knows the mulberry tree. The ... berries is delicious and has wonderful ...

ODE TO OLD SCHOOL SMOOTHIE

On any given day during the warmer months, this is what's in my cup. What I love about this blend is that the green juice and healthy fats get along so well. Using great fats with juice helps your body absorb all the nutrients from those important greens.

Makes 1 Serving

1½ cups favorite nonsweet green juice (see page 127 for juices)
½ avocado, pitted
1 tablespoon almond or coconut butter
3 ice cubes
1 teaspoon maca powder
½ teaspoon spirulina
1 cup spinach
3 drops Omica stevia
¼ pinch pink salt

Add all ingredients into a blender and blend on high for 1 minute.

Pour into your favorite smoothie glass and enjoy!

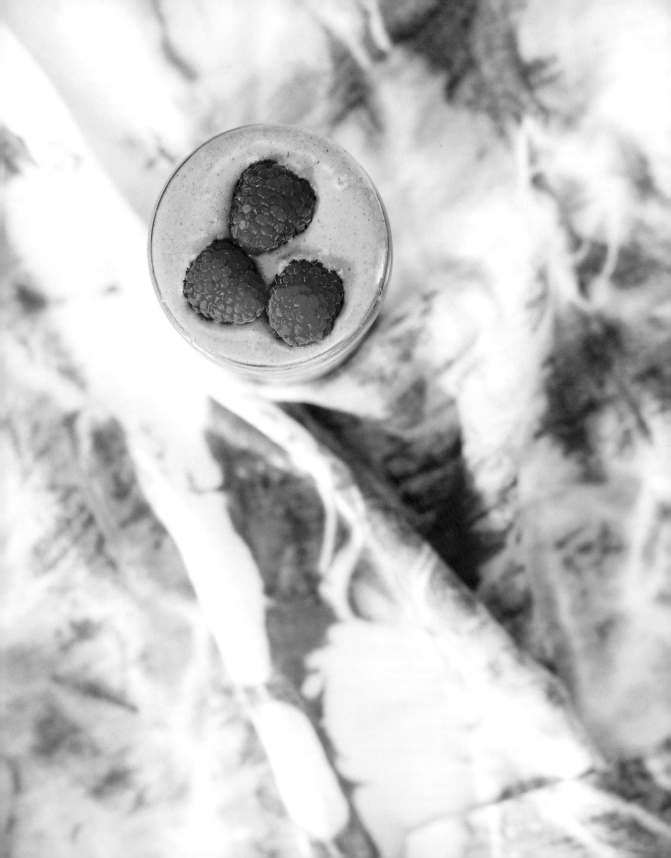

RASPBERRIES + CREAM SMOOTHIE

My son Henry requested that I add this recipe to the book. He loves this smoothie so much and thought you all would appreciate it. Very simple, and very delicious!

Makes 1 Serving

1½ cups favorite alternative milk
1 cup frozen raspberries
¾ cup young coconut meat
6 drops stevia or 3 dates, pitted
Pinch pink salt

Combine all the ingredients in a blender and blend on high until perfectly creamy.

Pour into your favorite smoothie glass and enjoy!

ORANGE CREAMCICLE

If you make nothing else in this book, make this. Creamy, dreamy orange float that will take you back to childhood summertimes. It's literally the yummiest thing ever. I have to give some credit here to my dear friend and longtime Local Juicery smoothie maker Douglas George. He had the idea to add this kind of smoothie to our menu, and while it's not official yet, if you come by, it's always on the "secret menu."

Makes 1 Serving

---

6 ounces almond milk or favorite
   alternative milk
6 ounces fresh squeezed orange
   juice
2 frozen bananas
1 scoop of your favorite protein
   powder
2 tablespoons stone-ground
   almond butter
¼ teaspoon pink salt

Combine all the ingredients in a blender and blend on high until perfectly creamy.

Pour into your favorite smoothie glass and enjoy!

NOTE: if you don't have oranges available, as sometimes it is hard to source organic ones, you can replace the orange juice with almond milk and add 3 to 5 drops of orange oil. I love Frontier or Simply Organic.

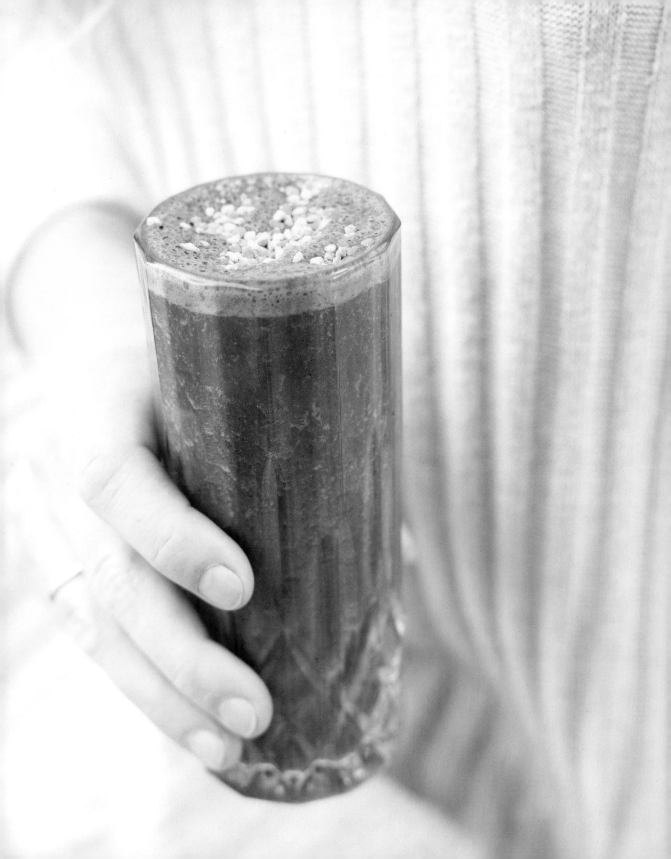

MAMA GAIA SMOOTHIE

This smoothie is a meal. It's loaded with incredibly filling and rich superfoods. Heart-healthy and fiber-rich kale, spinach, and flaxseed, antioxidants galore, a great source vitamin B_{12} thanks to the spirulina, and a nice push forward from cacao. I love this smoothie in the morning, especially when I'm in my ovulatory phase of my cycle (see more about that on page 41). It's supportive to hormones and provides everything you need to have a healthy start to your day.

Makes 1 Serving

2 cups almond milk or favorite
    alternative milk
1 banana, frozen, or 5 ice cubes
¼ medium avocado
1 cup spinach
1 cup kale
½ teaspoon spirulina
1 scoop of your favorite protein
1 teaspoon bee pollen
1 tablespoon almond butter
    (optional)
1 tablespoon raw cacao
1 tablespoon ground flaxseed
¼ teaspoon pink salt

Combine all the ingredients in a blender and blend on high until perfectly creamy.

Pour into your favorite smoothie glass and enjoy!

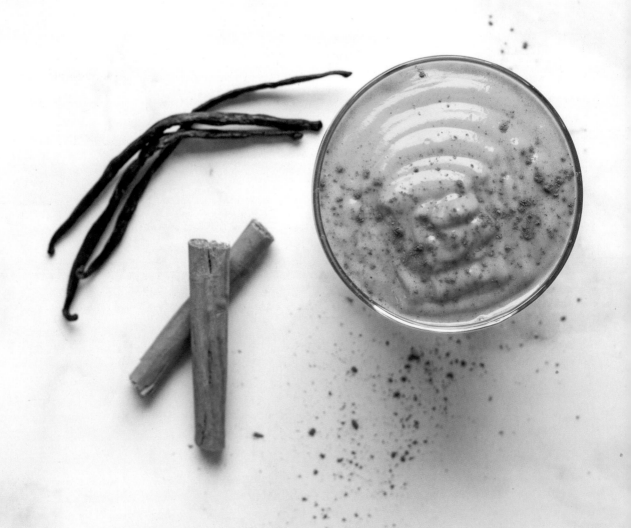

YAM BAM SMOOTHIE

Think autumn, but in dessert form. When the days still reach 90°F. but the nights and early mornings are crisp and cool. You know, that time when most of us start to crave the seasons' change. This smoothie is internally warming thanks to the spices. It's perfect for those between-season days. I've put a couple options here so you can make this smoothie work for your needs. I personally love maple syrup in my smoothies and typically will use it no matter what the experts say on glycemic load. It feeds my soul. But there are times (and my body will tell me) when I just need less sugar, so I opt for stevia, or just leave out the sweet entirely—the banana and sweet yam are typically sweet enough on their own. You can also replace the maple or stevia with your favorite go-to sweetener. I've given an option of using ice instead of banana for a lower glycemic version. I do recommend adding some kind of sweet if you omit the banana, though. Cinnamon is a wonderful blood sugar balancer as well being very high in antioxidants. It also has antifungal, anti-inflammatory, and antibacterial properties. Go ahead and pour heavy.

Makes 1 Serving

½ cup cooked sweet potato or
   yam, peeled
1 frozen banana, or 4 ice cubes
   (but will need more sweetener
   if you omit the banana)
2 cups almond milk (page 101)
½ teaspoon maca powder
⅛ teaspoon cardamom
⅛ teaspoon nutmeg
1 teaspoon maple syrup, or
   4 drops Omica vanilla stevia
1 tablespoon stone-ground
   almond butter
¼ teaspoon pink salt

Combine all the ingredients in a blender and blend on high until perfectly creamy.

Pour into your favorite smoothie glass and top with cinnamon, snap a picture, and enjoy!

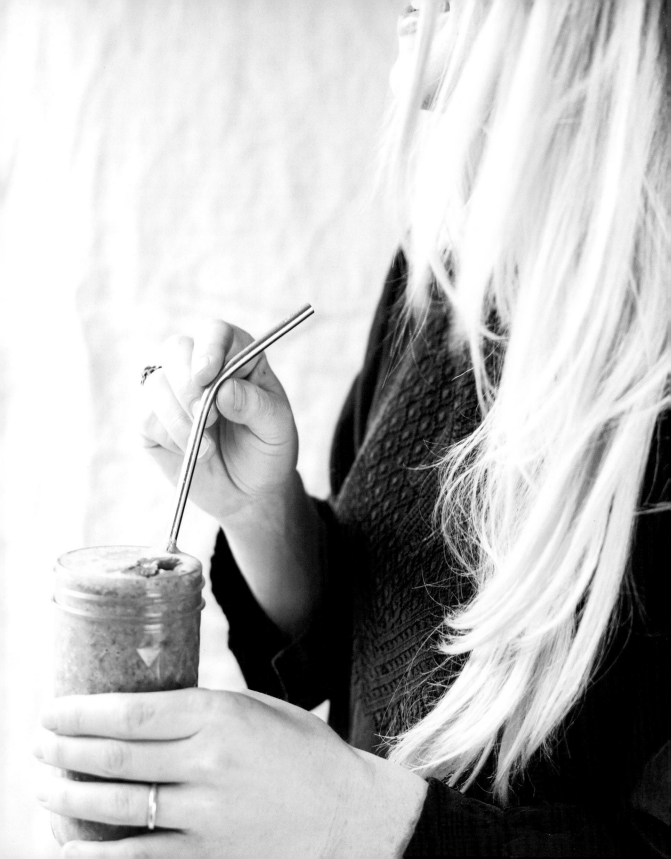

CILANTRO DETOX SHAKE

I drink a version of this at least two days a week. It's an incredible heavy-metal cleanser and helps make your system more alkaline, setting you up for a day of energy. Cilantro is a powerful heavy-metal cleanser, and I think it should be incorporated into every meal in some way. Most of us live in areas with dense population and poor air quality, we are also bombarded by Wi-Fi and cell phone radiation all day long. This shake helps neutralize some of the damage that our modern life can inflict.

Makes 1 Serving

2 cups fresh orange juice
1 bunch cilantro
1 teaspoon fresh ginger, minced
½ frozen banana or frozen
  avocado
Pinch of pink salt

Combine all the ingredients in a blender and blend on high until perfectly creamy.

Pour into your favorite smoothie glass and enjoy!

TROPICANA

Basically a beach vacation in your cup. I used avocado in this recipe instead of banana for a little bit of a creamier texture and less glycemic load. This is actually something you can do with all of these recipes. You can use ½ avocado and 3–5 ice cubes to replace two frozen bananas, just be aware that the sweet ratio may be off and need some balancing. You can use dates or stevia depending on your needs.

Makes 1 Serving

2 cups fresh coconut water or
  almond milk
1 large handful spinach
¼ frozen avocado
2 dates, pitted
1 tablespoon coconut oil
½ cup frozen or fresh mango
1 cup fresh or frozen pineapple
1 teaspoon fresh ginger, minced
¼ teaspoon pink salt

Combine all the ingredients in a blender and blend on high until perfectly creamy.

Pour into your favorite smoothie glass and enjoy!

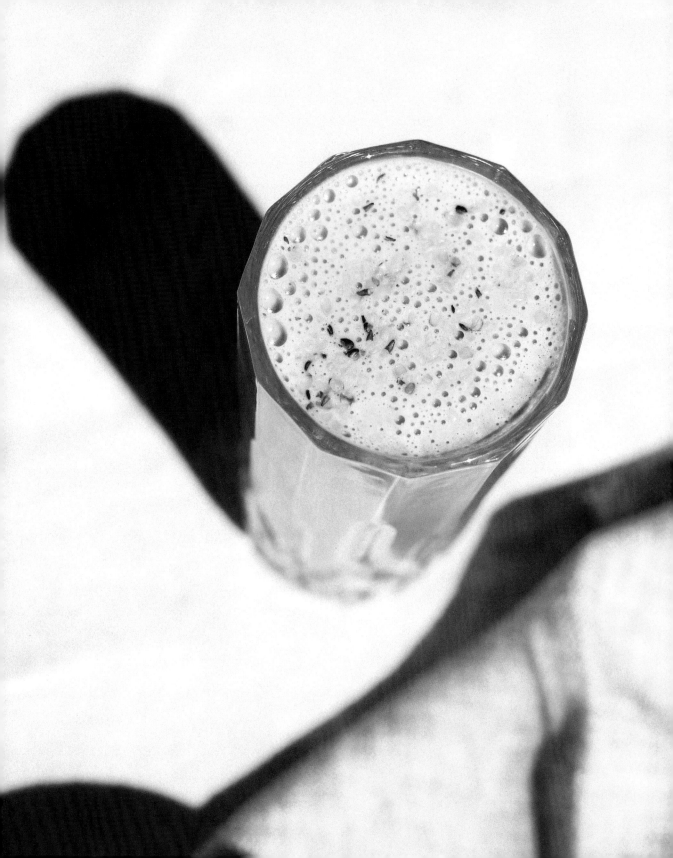

A STRAWBERRY SMOOTHIE

I crave this smoothie in the summertime. I had a two-month stint where all I drank at Local Juicery (my café) was this. I literally made 32 ounces of it every day. The strawberries offer incredible vitamin C, while the maca works hard at balancing your hormones. My little boy loves his version of this smoothie, too, but for him I use a little cacao instead of the maca. Maca is best for adults since children are still developing. I never give children or young teens maca just to be on the safe side.

Makes 1 Serving

2 cups almond milk or favorite alternative milk
1½ cup frozen strawberries
1 scoop of your favorite protein powder
½ teaspoon maca powder
2 tablespoons stone-ground almond butter
¼ teaspoon pink salt

Combine all the ingredients in a blender and blend on high until perfectly creamy.

Pour into your favorite smoothie glass and enjoy!

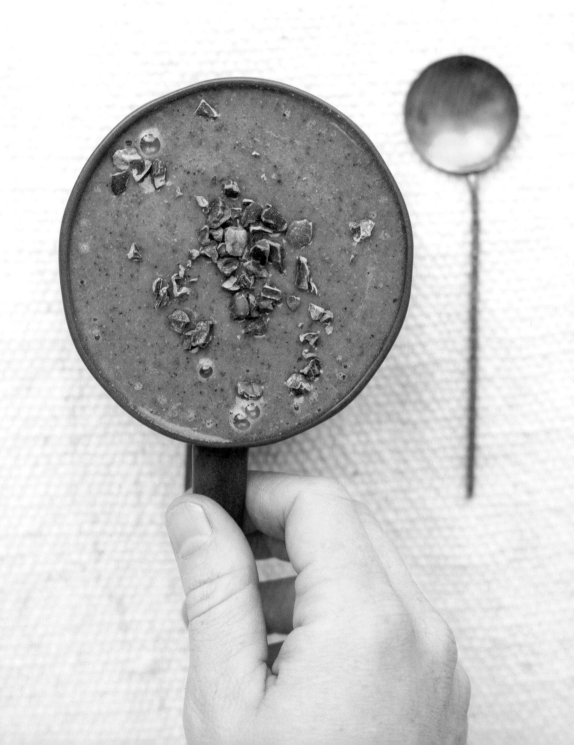

MINTY MAGIC

Think mint chocolate chip ice-cream but healthy, like really, really healthy. My son, who is five years old, is obsessed with this and with the amount of spinach and spirulina in it, I'm happy to give it to him whenever! Spirulina is amazing for vegans because of its naturally occurring vitamin B_{12} and the spinach is loaded with iron which vegans are in need of too. The cacao nibs give a little crunch, which is fun when you need a texture variation. I love this as a quick on-the-go lunch option when I don't have time to make a full meal. You can substitute avocado and a couple ice cubes for the banana to make it lower glycemic.

Makes 1 Serving

2 frozen bananas, or ½ avocado
plus 5 ice cubes
14 ounces almond milk
(page 101)
1 tablespoon of your favorite
protein powder (optional)
2 heaping handfuls spinach
1 teaspoon spirulina
2 dates, pitted
2 full droppers mint oil (frontier
organics is my favorite)
2 tablespoons stone-ground
almond butter
Squeeze of lemon
¼ teaspoon pink salt
2 tablespoons cacao nibs

Combine all the ingredients except cacao nibs in a blender and blend on high until perfectly creamy.

Pour into your favorite smoothie glass and top with cacao nibs and enjoy!

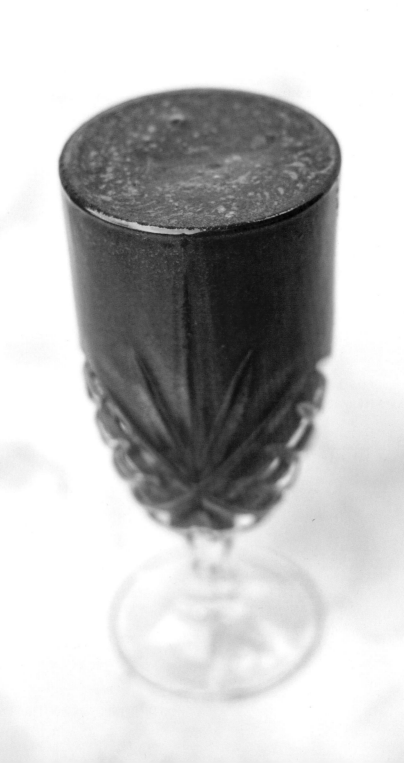

RED VELVET MYLKSHAKE

This no-guilt dessert is creamy and rich, but still leaves you feeling energized and light. It's great for a summertime evening dessert. The beet from the juice makes it the perfect deep red velvet color. If you want a low-glycemic version, try using a frozen avocado and a couple ice cubes in place of the banana. You can sweeten with stevia if need be. This smoothie is great as ice cream too! To make, use 6 ounces of juice and let the banana be the cream. You'll need a high-speed blender for making ice cream, but the result is worth it. Make sure you have a plunger when making extra thick smoothies or ice creams.

Makes 1 Serving

---

2 cups Rooty Juice (page 131)
2 frozen bananas
3 tablespoons raw cacao powder
2 tablespoons stone-ground
   almond butter
½ teaspoon vanilla extract
¼ teaspoon pink salt

Combine all the ingredients in a blender and blend on high until perfectly creamy.

Pour into your favorite smoothie glass and enjoy!

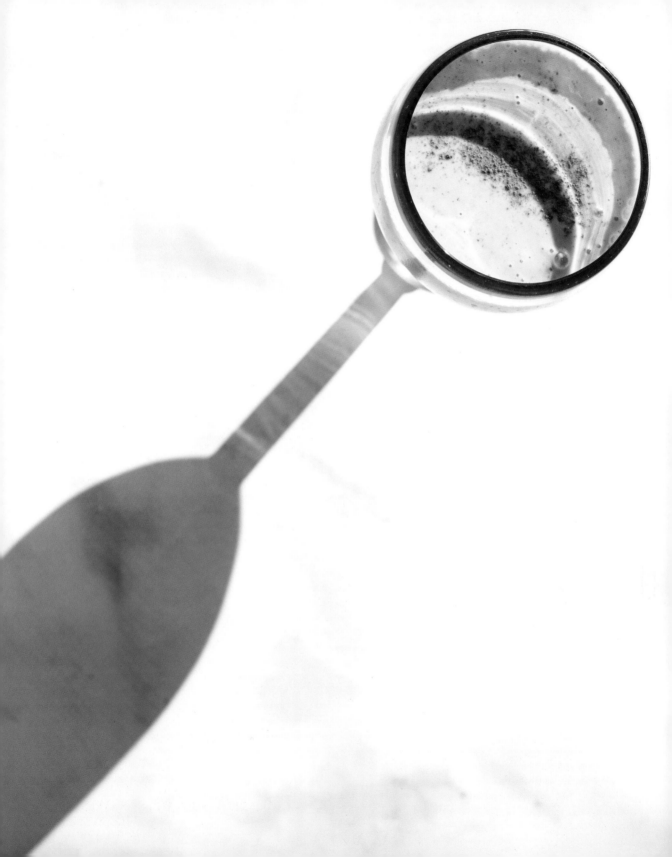

DATE SHAKE

Sometimes you just need something that's comforting and delicious, and this is your shake for that time. You can really elaborate on this shake and make it even more dynamic by adding cacao, protein, maca, or any of your favorite superfoods. I kept this recipe simple because I really love the vanilla flavor that comes out, but feel free to play with it and make it your own.
Makes 1 Serving

1 frozen banana
1 cup ice
14 ounces almond milk (page 101)
3 dates, pitted
2 tablespoons stone-ground
   almond butter
¼ teaspoon vanilla bean powder
¼ teaspoon cinnamon
¼ teaspoon pink salt

Combine all the ingredients in a blender and blend on high until perfectly creamy.

Pour into your favorite smoothie glass and enjoy!

AVOCADO CACAO SHAKE

A simple and classic shake. I've always loved it. I've played with a few other variations, sometimes adding almond extract, sometimes omitting the avocado and making it more of a slushy, sometimes adding banana for a super dreamy creamy milkshake. However you do it, it's good! You can also add your favorite protein and make it a meal!
Makes 1 Serving

14 ounces almond or favorite
   alternative milk (page 101)
½ avocado
4 ice cubes
1 tablespoon stone-ground
   almond butter
2 tablespoons raw cacao powder
1 teaspoon maca powder
2 teaspoons maple syrup or
   4 drops Omica stevia
¼ teaspoon pink salt

Combine all the ingredients in a blender and blend on high until perfectly creamy.

Pour into your favorite smoothie glass and enjoy!

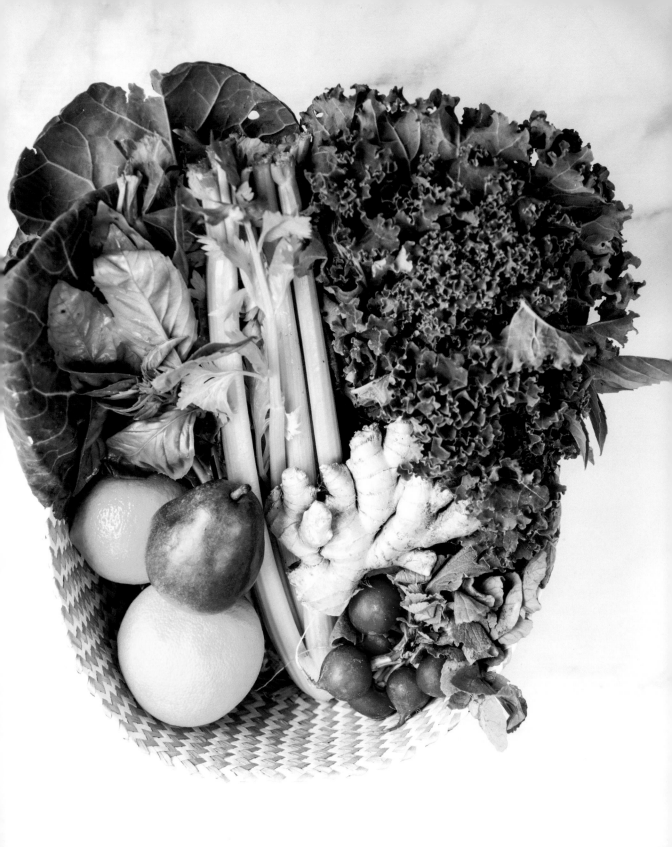

JUICES

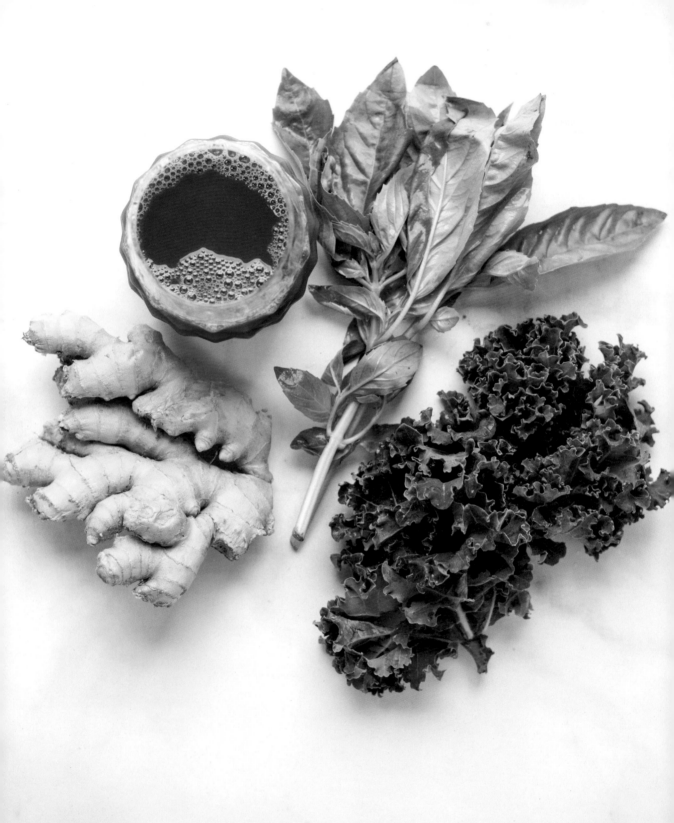

SIMPLE GREENS

Sometimes the best things are the simplest things. Getting too complex can hide some of the amazing natural flavors that come from fruits and vegetables. This is one of my go-to juices, I switch up the greens depending on what I have in the house, but it's always based on this. The lemon gives it a well-rounded flavor, and the ginger gives it a nice kick. You can use any citrus and play with other options like jalapeño or turmeric in place of the ginger. Get creative!

Makes 2 Servings

---

2 green apples
2 cucumbers, peeled or well
   washed
1 bunch kale
3 cups spinach, packed tightly
1 large thumb ginger
½ lemon, peeled

Wash and chop all ingredients and send through your juicer.

Pour into a glass and enjoy!

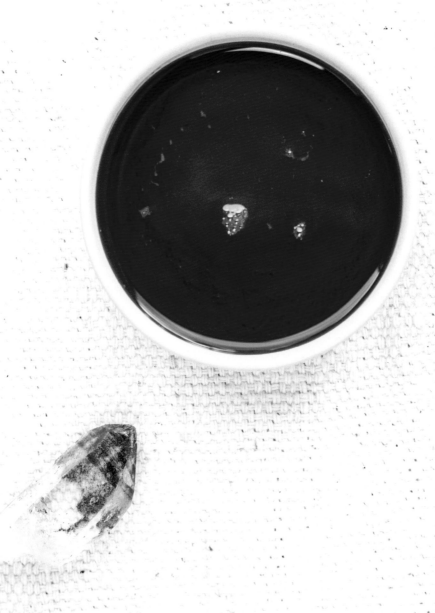

ROOTY

Talk about delicious, this juice could be dessert. It's so yummy! I actually use it as a base to a fun smoothie (see page 123). Beyond the flavor, it is also incredibly healing—it helps support the immune system and lowers inflammation in the body while also gently detoxing your liver. Additionally, it's high in Vitamin A and folate! If you're having troubles with your digestion, this is the juice for you.

Makes 2 Servings

---

1 beet, peeled and quartered
2 green apples
6 carrots, quartered
2 large thumbs turmeric
1 large thumb ginger

Wash and chop all ingredients and send through your juicer.

Pour into a glass and enjoy!

HERBS + GREENS

I love the way the herbs come together to make a really fun and dynamic flavor profile in this juice. If you like a little sweet, you can add one green apple and still keep the glycemic index low. I use a cold press in place of a juice and find that this creates the creamiest and most delicious juices. If you're a new mom, this juice is great for postpartum. The fennel supports a steady flow of breast milk!

Makes 2 Servings

---

4 cups spinach
4 large green chard leaves
4 celery stalks
2 cucumbers, quartered
2 cups mint
1 cup cilantro
1 cup basil
1 fennel bulb
1 thumb ginger
1 lemon, peeled

Wash and chop all ingredients and send through your juicer.

Pour into a glass and enjoy!

SUMMER GREENS

Juicing is amazing. With today's industry-funded studies and overwhelm of health options, it can be highly confusing when trying to decide what's right for one's body. I always recommend going as close to the earth as possible. Juice, when cold pressed or fresh, is one of the most detoxifying, alkalizing, and nutritious healing potions out there. I personally only drink cold pressed raw juice but making it in an at-home juicer is fine so long as you are consuming the juice within minutes of juicing it. This is where some of the confusion with juice starts—when juice just sits there or is stored (if it's not cold-pressed) then the juice quickly turns to glucose, but if you sip it right away, you are getting amazing nutritional benefits.

Makes 2 Servings

---

2 large handfuls spinach
1 bunch kale
2 cucumbers, peeled
½ ripe pineapple
1 head romaine lettuce
1 green apple

Wash all fruits, vegetables, and leafy greens. Juice all ingredients, starting with the spinach and kale, and following with the cucumbers. This helps push greens through.

Pour into your favorite tall glass enjoy! Best to drink within 5 minutes of juicing unless you are using a cold-press or masticating juicer.

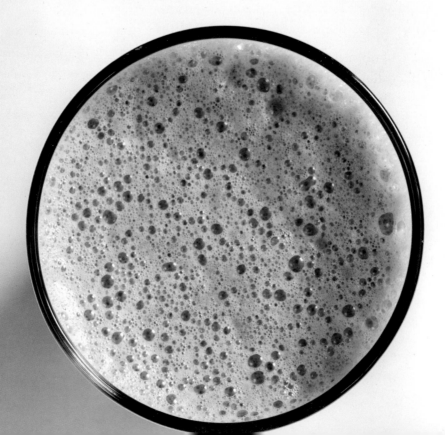

SOMETHING GOLDEN

I love the tart but sweet quality to this juice, it's simple but potent. You don't need much to make magic when you're using mother nature's amazing foods. The turmeric and ginger give you an amazing immune boost while the lemon and pineapple energize and alkalize.

Makes 2 Servings

1 whole ripe pineapple, cut into
   small pieces
1½ lemons
1 (3-inch) piece fresh ginger
1 (2-inch) piece fresh turmeric

NOTE: Blend a banana into this for an epic smoothie!

Wash all fruits and roots.

Peel the lemons before juicing or juice with a citrus press separately.

Juice all ingredients, starting with some pineapple and adding in the roots in between.

Pour into your favorite tall glass and enjoy! Best to drink within 5 minutes of juicing unless you are using a cold-press or masticating juicer.

CILANTRO PUNCH

Cilantro is one of my most favorite healing foods. I like to put it in as many creations as possible. It's an incredibly potent heavy-metal detoxifier. We are constantly bombarded by metals daily, from our air and water and even foods. This juice will work hard to help remove these toxins and support you with minerals and hydration.

Makes 2 Servings

1 lime, juiced
8 stalks celery
1 cucumber, quartered
2 cups tightly packed cilantro
2 green apples, quartered

Wash all fruits, vegetables, and greens.

Peel the lime before juicing or juice with a citrus press separately.

Juice all ingredients.

Pour into your favorite tall glass and enjoy! Best to drink within 5 minutes of juicing unless you are using a cold-press or masticating juicer.

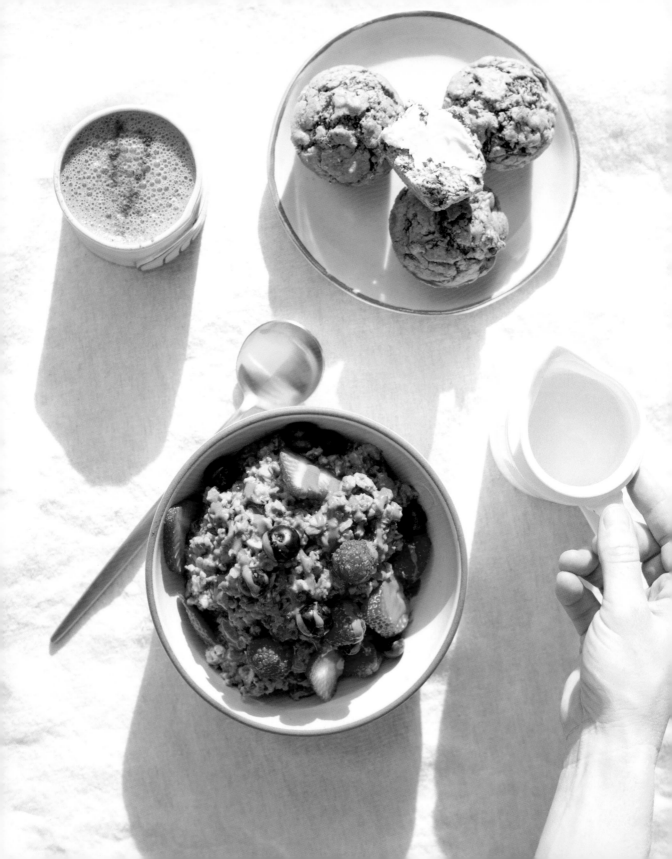

BREAKFAST

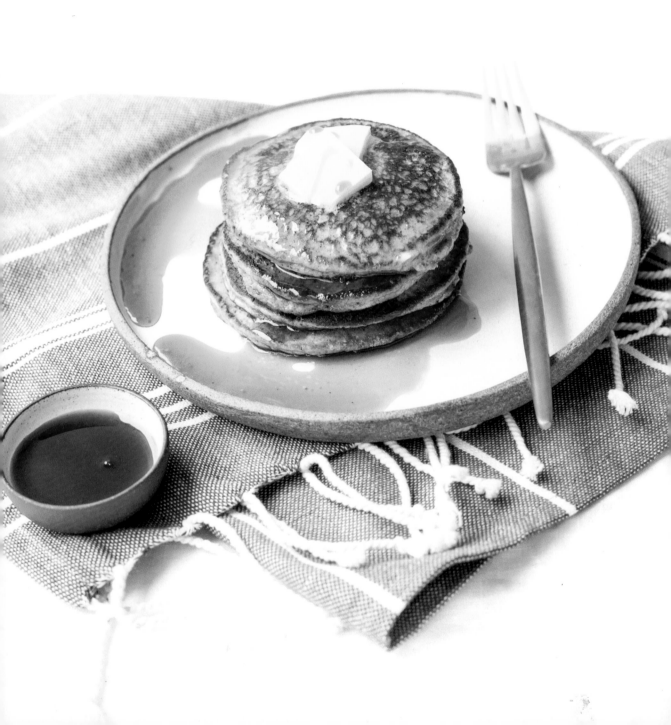

PROTEIN PANCAKES

I made this recipe for my son because I wanted to get good nutrition in him while still making something that he'd love. It's a win-win recipe. I love it too. The psyllium and flax add great fiber to our diet and the spinach and banana add in wonderful power nutrient boosts. Another wonderful thing about this recipe is all you need is a blender to make it!

Makes About 8 Pancakes

---

2 large bananas
¼ cup alternative milk
6 farm-fresh eggs
3 tablespoons flax seed
2 tablespoons psyllium husk
1 cup gluten-free oats
1 teaspoon reishi powder
  (optional)
½ teaspoon pink salt
1 teaspoon vanilla extract
Ghee or coconut oil for the skillet

In a blender combine banana, milk, eggs, flax, psyllium, oats, reishi, salt, and vanilla. Blend until well combined and green from the spinach.

Heat the skillet with ghee or coconut oil, and pour three 3-inch pancakes into the pan.

Once the bubbles are on the sides and middle, they are ready to flip. These pancakes require about 1 minute per side once the pan is hot.

Top with delightful goodness and enjoy!

NOTE: You can add a couple handfuls of spinach to this recipe to make it even healthier!

APPLE FRITTER PANCAKES

This recipe is inspired by my dear friend's grandmother, a traditional Italian grandmother, and I was lucky enough to be included in some breakfasts at their home when I was a child. This recipe always stuck with me. This is my version of her classic.

Makes About 12 Pancakes

---

3 apples
3 cups oat flour
½ cup brown rice flour
3 tablespoons psyllium husk
1 teaspoon salt
½ teaspoon baking soda
½ teaspoon baking powder
½ cup coconut sugar
7 eggs
2 tablespoons coconut oil, melted
¼ cup oat or almond milk
Butter or ghee for greasing your pan

NOTE: These save really well! Make ahead of time and pop in the toaster when ready to eat.

Cut your three apples in small pieces that can fit though a food processor feeder. Remove the S blade and attach the shredder on your food processor. Once shredded, use a nut milk bag or cheesecloth to strain out the liquid from the apples. Make sure to save the liquid in a bowl.

After the liquid is removed, place the shreds in a large bowl.

Pour the apple juice into another bowl, and set aside.

Add the oat flour, brown rice four, psyllium husk, salt, baking soda, baking powder, and coconut sugar into the shredded apples. Mix until well combined.

Add the eggs, melted coconut oil, and almond milk into the apple juice. Whisk until well combined.

Grease your pan with butter or ghee. Once it's ready, pour ¼ cup of mix per pancake.

Once bubbles appear around and in the middle of the cake, it's ready to flip! Cook about a minute and a half per side.

Top with cinnamon, butter, and whatever else you adore!

RASPBERRY CHIA PUDDING + CORDYCEPS CARAMEL

This recipe is decadent and healthy, featuring heart-healthy chia, protein-filled almond butter, and master immune booster and adaptogen cordyceps mushroom powder. Perfect for a leisurely weekend brunch. You can also omit the caramel and make this recipe ahead of time. Chia pudding can be the best on-the-go breakfast. Since the seeds expand, they help keep you feeling fuller for longer.

Makes 2 Servings

chia pudding

1 cup raspberries, fresh or frozen
1 cup alternative milk (page 101)
2 tablespoons stone-ground almond butter
¼ teaspoon vanilla extract or powder
1 tablespoon maple syrup or 4 drops Omica stevia
5 drops rose essence
¼ teaspoon pink salt
5 tablespoons chia seeds

raspberry cordyceps caramel topping

¼ cup stone-ground almond butter
3–5 tablespoons water
¼ cup defrosted frozen raspberries
½ teaspoon cordyceps mushroom powder
2 tablespoons maple syrup or 3 drops Omica stevia
Squeeze of lemon
¼ teaspoon pink salt

make the chia pudding: If you're using frozen raspberries, let them defrost.

Blend together milk, almond butter, vanilla, maple syrup or stevia, rose essence, and salt until well combined.

Pour into a bowl and add in chia. Whisk together. Put the mixture in the refrigerator to set (about 20 to 30 minutes).

Once it has set up into a Jell-O-like consistency, fold in the raspberries.

Top with raspberry caramel, more raspberries, or fresh roses for a beautiful display.

make the topping: In a small bowl combine almond butter, water, raspberries, cordyceps, sweetener, lemon, and salt. Whisk until caramel is ready for pouring.

Drizzle on top of the pudding. Snap a photo and serve.

> **NOTE:** The chia base can be made the night before. It keeps wonderfully!

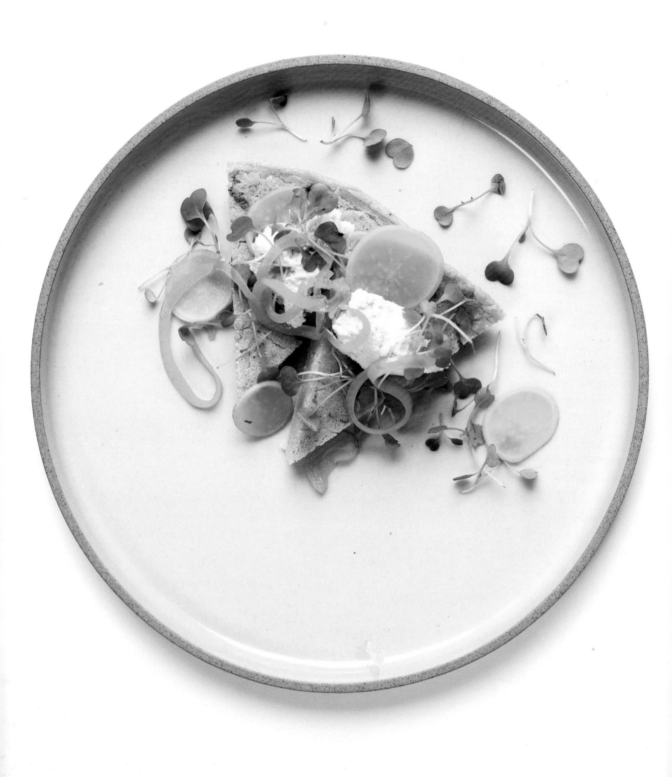

SAVORY SOCCA PANCAKES

Socca is amazing–I could eat this every day. It's a traditional French food (popular in Nice) and is known as a street food. There is an Italian version that is very similar called *farinata*. This recipe is gluten-free, full of fiber and protein, 100 percent plant-based, but gives you the feeling you're enjoying an omelet or very glutenous bread. I like it savory, topped with cashew cheese, pesto, or even hummus, but you can also make a more sweet version adding cinnamon in place of the herbs and maybe a little maple syrup. Enjoy!

Makes 4 Servings

---

socca
2 cups chickpea flour
2 cups almond milk (page 101)
1½ tablespoons melted coconut
   oil, plus extra for oiling the pan
1 teaspoon pink salt
1 teaspoon ground black pepper
1 tablespoon chives, minced
1 tablespoon parsley, minced
1 teaspoon cumin (optional)

toppers
Macadamia nut butter (page 261)
Turmeric and radish pickles
   (page 255)
Microgreens

In a large bowl, combine the chickpea flour, milk, oil, salt, pepper, herbs, and cumin. Whisk until well blended. Let it sit for 30 minutes or up to one hour to set.

Preheat your pan! Do this by preheating your oven to 450°F and letting your skillet warm for 10 minutes (make sure no oil is in it yet).

Remove the skillet from the oven and place on the stove top (make sure to place the handle away from yourself). Add oil to the bottom and rub a bit on the sides with a paper towel. Pour the batter into the center of your pan. Use a spoon to help cover the entire surface of the pan.

Put back into the oven and cook for about 20 minutes. If it is expanding too quickly, move to a lower rack.

Use a spatula to work the socca and remove it from the pan onto a nice plate or cutting board. You can cut into squares or pie cuts. Top with herbs or a simple cashew cheese (see page 261).

NOTE: You can use lentil flour for this recipe as well. You can also ferment the mixture on your countertop for up to two days. I tried this but prefer it without the heavy ferment.

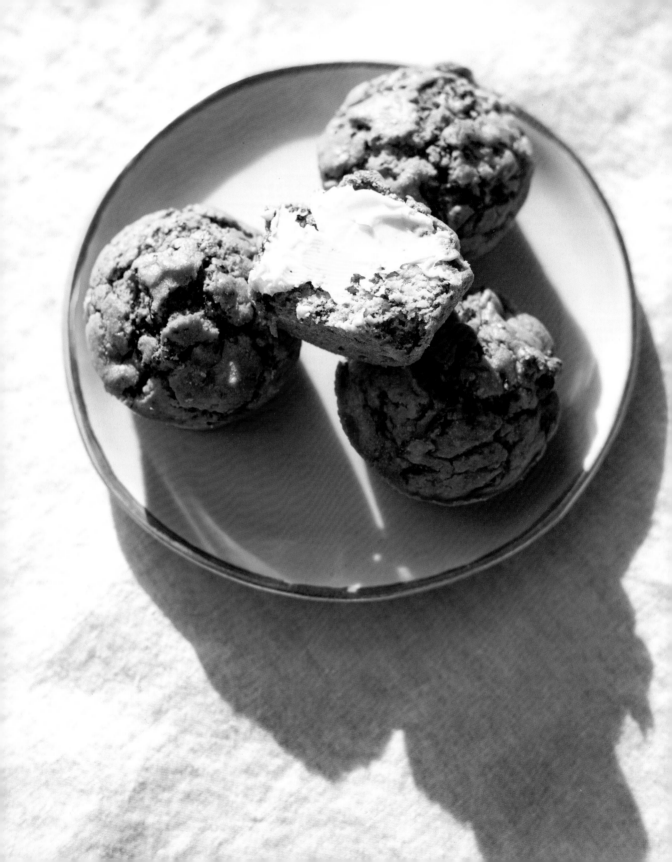

LEAN GREEN CHICKPEA MUFFINS

I love having savory breakfasts. So often we load up on sweets, and our blood sugar goes nuts—no wonder we're tired by lunch. Try this high-protein savory muffin for a change. I bet you'll be lasting all day long! Great for children too. I pack these in my little guy's lunch and he loves them. Get the greens in wherever you can!

Makes 12 Muffins

---

2 cups spinach, tightly packed and chopped
1 cup lightly steamed broccoli, chopped
Coconut oil
2 cups chickpea flour
1 tablespoon chives, minced
¼ cup nutritional yeast
1 teaspoon baking soda
½ teaspoon pink salt
1 teaspoon black pepper
1 tablespoon coconut oil
2 eggs
1 tablespoon maple syrup
1½ cups almond milk (page 101)

Preheat oven to 400°F.

Sauté spinach and steamed broccoli in a little coconut oil for about 5 minutes. Set aside.

In a bowl, combine chickpea flour, chives, nutritional yeast, baking soda, pink salt, and black pepper.

In a separate bowl combine coconut oil, eggs, maple syrup, and almond milk. Add sautéed vegetables to the wet mix. Stir until well combined.

Brush muffin tin with coconut oil or use muffin cups. Fill cups with ¼ cup chickpea batter.

Bake for 20 minutes. You'll know they're ready when a toothpick inserted in the center comes out clean.

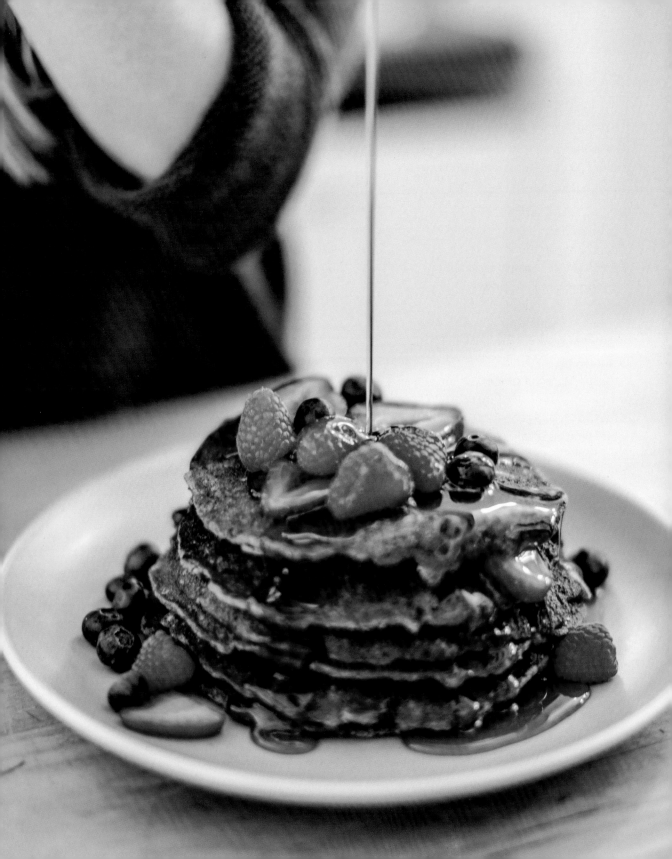

BANANA BUCKWHEAT FLAPJACKS

The only banana pancake recipe you'll ever need. Vegan, delicious, and Instagram-worthy. I top these with so many fun things. My favorite indulgence is topping with peanut butter, bananas, and maple syrup. I don't know if anything gets better than that.

Makes 8 Pancakes

1 cup buckwheat flour
1 cup oat flour
1 cup almond flour
1½ teaspoons baking soda
½ teaspoon baking powder
1 cup coconut sugar
1 teaspoon salt
¼ cup arrowroot
1 teaspoon cinnamon
⅓ cup chia seeds or 2 eggs if not
   making vegan
2 medium bananas
1 tablespoon apple cider vinegar
3 tablespoons vanilla
1 tablespoon coconut oil, melted
½ cup almond milk

In a bowl combine buckwheat flour, oat flour, almond flour, baking soda, baking powder, coconut sugar, salt, arrowroot, and cinnamon. Whisk so that it is all well combined.

Then in a blender combine chia seed or eggs, bananas, vinegar, vanilla, coconut oil, and almond milk. Blend until smooth.

Pour wet mix into the dry mix and mix well.

Pour about ¼ cup of batter into a hot skillet that is oiled with coconut oil or ghee, cook until the middle of the cake begins to bubble, and then flip. You should cook about 2 minutes on each side.

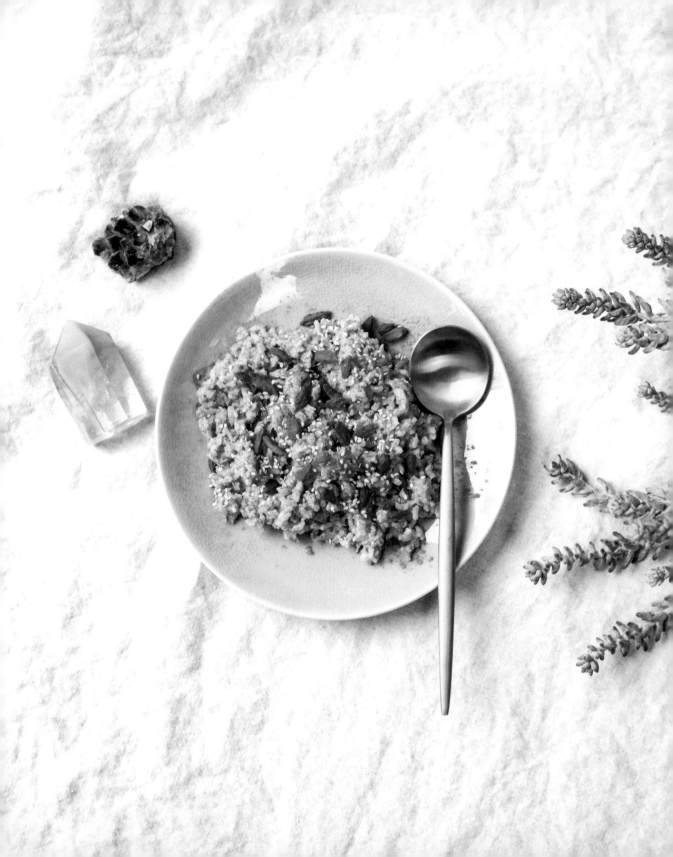

TAHINI + SPROUTED RICE PORRIDGE

This recipe was passed down to me from my mother. One of the three recipes she's ever really shared (or made, for that matter). My mother is many things, but a cook is not one of them. I was basically raised on Annie's frozen pizza and potpies. Bless her. She knew how important food was but was a single mother hustling to get her business launched and trying to raise me. She did the best she could when it came to food, and whenever she did cook, I loved it so much. I specifically remember eating this porridge on cold winter mornings. The tahini creates a wonderful savory flavor, and the maple, well, it just makes everything awesome.

Makes 1 Serving

---

1 cup precooked sprouted rice (see page 251 for the perfect rice)

2 tablespoons tahini

3 teaspoons maple syrup or 4 drops Omica stevia

¼ teaspoon cinnamon

¼ teaspoon pink salt

In a small saucepan add rice, tahini, maple syrup, cinnamon, and salt. Warm up to desired temperature and then pour into a bowl. Top with favorite toppings.

NOTE: You can add fun things like walnuts, raisins, or goji berries to this porridge. I actually love toasted pumpkin seeds on it! Whatever your heart desires.

MONDAY OATS

Simple and quick, exactly what most of us need come Monday morning. You'll get the good omega fatty acids from the flax and chia as well as the added healthy fiber. Great for your brain and your heart! The coconut oil pushes the flavor and texture to the next level. Sweeten however you please, and top with extra berries if you can spare some time.

Makes 2 Servings

---

1 cup sprouted oats
2 cups walnut or almond milk
  (page 101)
¾ cup frozen berries of choice
½ teaspoon pink salt
¼ cup ground flaxseed
1 tablespoon chia seeds
1 tablespoon coconut oil
Sweetener of choice

Combine oats, milk, berries, and salt in a saucepan. Bring to a boil, then turn to low. Simmer the oatmeal for around 20 minutes until very soft.

Stir in the flax, chia seeds, and coconut oil, and sweeten to taste.

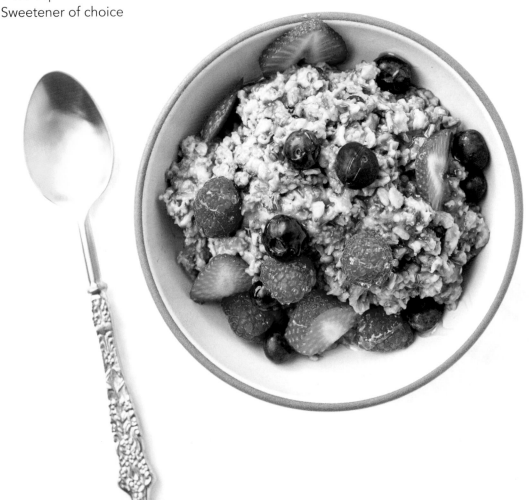

BANANA BUCKWHEAT MUFFINS

Buckwheat is actually one of my favorite seeds. It gives you that desired grain texture but without the inflammation. You can make buckwheat the same way you would oatmeal (see page 149 for a great recipe); it works wonderfully as a morning porridge. This muffin recipe is very simple, but tastes like you spent a day in the kitchen! The walnuts are a wonderful addition for extra brainpower and healthy fats. Enjoy these muffins as a quick grab-and-go breakfast when you don't have time for a full meal. Try a little coconut oil or raw butter on one when it's hot out of the oven, maybe a little drizzle of raw honey . . . delicious.

Makes 12 Muffins

½ cup buckwheat flour
½ cup almond flour
1 teaspoon baking soda
1 teaspoon pink salt
1 cup walnuts, crushed (optional)
2 ripe bananas, mashed
1 cup maple syrup
3 tablespoons coconut oil, melted
2 eggs or chia eggs (page 253)
1 tablespoon vanilla
1 teaspoon almond extract

Preheat oven to 350°F.

In metal bowl, combine all dry ingredients, stirring well.

In a blender combine banana, maple syrup, oil, eggs, vanilla, and almond extract.

Add the wet mix to the dry ingredients and mix very well until everything is well combined and dough becomes thick.

Line a muffin tin with muffin cups, and divide the mixture between them. Bake for 20 minutes or until a toothpick inserted in the center comes out clean.

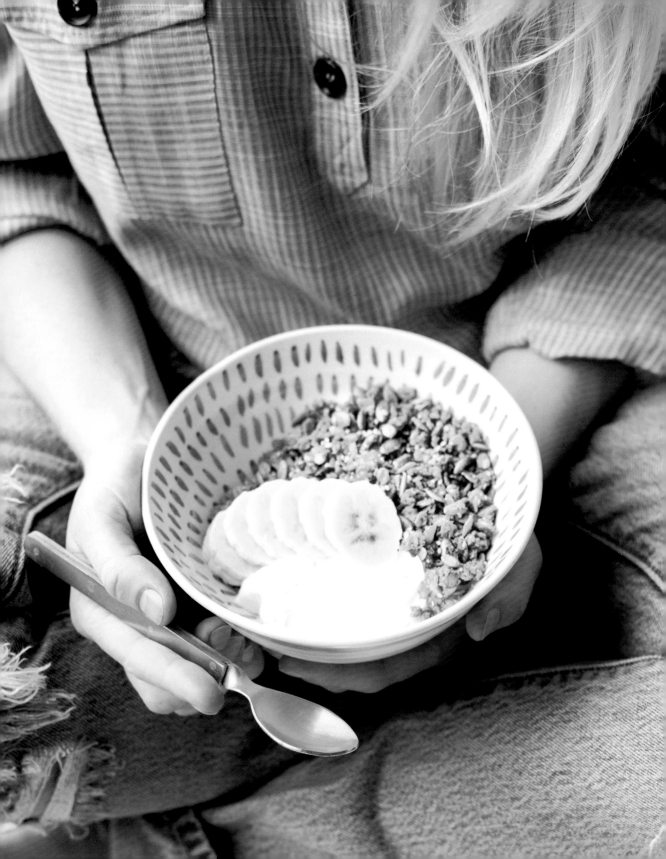

TURMERIC + PEPITA GRANOLA

I quit buying granola a long time ago. Every time I would read the ingredients I was let down. Either sunflower oil, canola oil, sugar, or some other additive that I would rather do without. Making your own granola is so easy, and the flavor options are endless. I love turmeric for all its healing qualities, I also love its amazing color! This granola pairs wonderfully with the coconut yogurt on page 161.

Makes 6 Servings

---

2 cups pepitas
2 cups sprouted oats
1 cup almond flour
½ cup sesame seeds
¾ cup maple syrup
¾ cup coconut oil
2 tablespoons vanilla extract
2 tablespoons turmeric powder
1 teaspoon salt
1 teaspoon cinnamon
½ teaspoon ginger

Preheat the oven to 350°F.

In a large bowl, combine pepitas, sprouted oats, almond flour, and sesame seeds. Stir and set aside.

In a high-speed blender, combine maple syrup, coconut oil, vanilla, turmeric powder, salt, cinnamon, and ginger. Blend until well combined.

Pour wet mix into the dry mix and mash with your hands.

Line a baking sheet with parchment paper and spread mix onto it evenly. Bake for 35 minutes or until golden brown; check frequently, as it can burn easily.

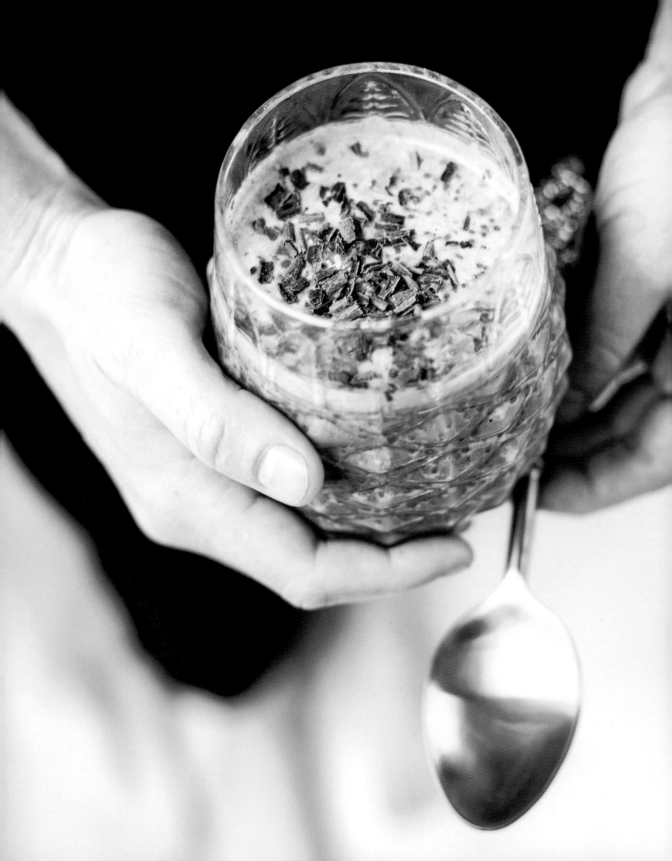

CHOCOLATE HAZELNUT CHIA

Simple and so rewarding. There's something magical that happens when you pair hazelnuts with chocolate. This is like eating dessert for breakfast, but it's incredibly healthy. Win-win! I ate this all though my pregnancy and continue to enjoy it now. I love it topped with a whole lotta berries and bananas and a good healthy portion of almond butter! By the way, when you're eating a plant-inspired diet full of healthy vegetables, fruits, seeds, nuts, and grains, you can have a good-sized portion of healthy fats like almond butter without any worries. Your body loves it.

Makes 2 Servings

---

3 cups hazelnut milk (page 103)
1 cup raw cacao powder
½ teaspoon salt
1 teaspoon vanilla
1 tablespoon maca
3 tablespoons maple syrup
1 cup chia seeds

Pour hazelnut milk into your blender.

Add in cacao powder, salt, vanilla, maca, and maple syrup. Blend until well combined.

In a bowl, combine chia and chocolate milk mixture. Whisk and then place in the refrigerator, whisking every 10 minutes or so.

Once it has sat for 30 minutes it should be ready to eat! It's fine to let this sit overnight as well.

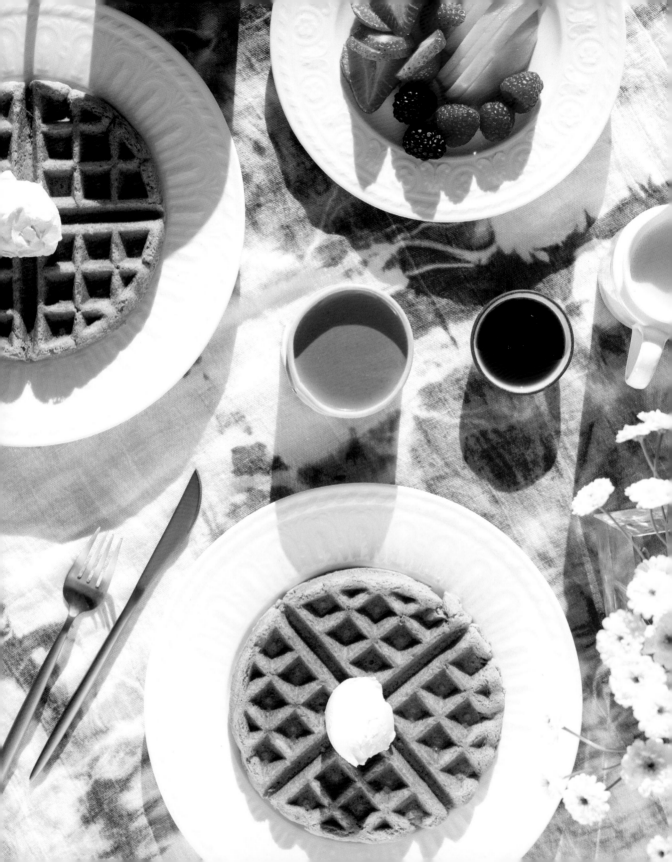

MATCHA WAFFLE

Matcha is something I am incredibly fond of. It's light, energizing, and antioxidant-rich. It's one of my top three favorite superfoods. The color makes it so fun to add to waffles! Try serving with stone-ground almond butter and maple syrup! Simply amazing. I've also added a vegan version that substitutes chia for eggs.

Makes About 8 Waffles

2½ cups almond flour
1 cup brown rice flour
¼ cup arrowroot
1 teaspoon baking soda
4 eggs or chia eggs (page 253)
1 teaspoon salt
¼ cup maple syrup
⅓ cup coconut oil, melted
1½ cups almond milk
1½ cups spinach, packed tightly
3 tablespoons matcha powder

In a bowl, combine almond flour, brown rice flour, arrowroot, and baking soda. Stir well and set aside.

In a Vitamix combine egg or chia, salt, maple syrup, coconut oil, almond milk, spinach, and matcha. Blend well until very creamy.

Pour wet mix into reserved dry mix. Whisk until combined.

Heat waffle iron, then pour in ½ cup (or suggested amount) of batter per waffle maker instructions until cooked.

Top with your favorite toppings and enjoy.

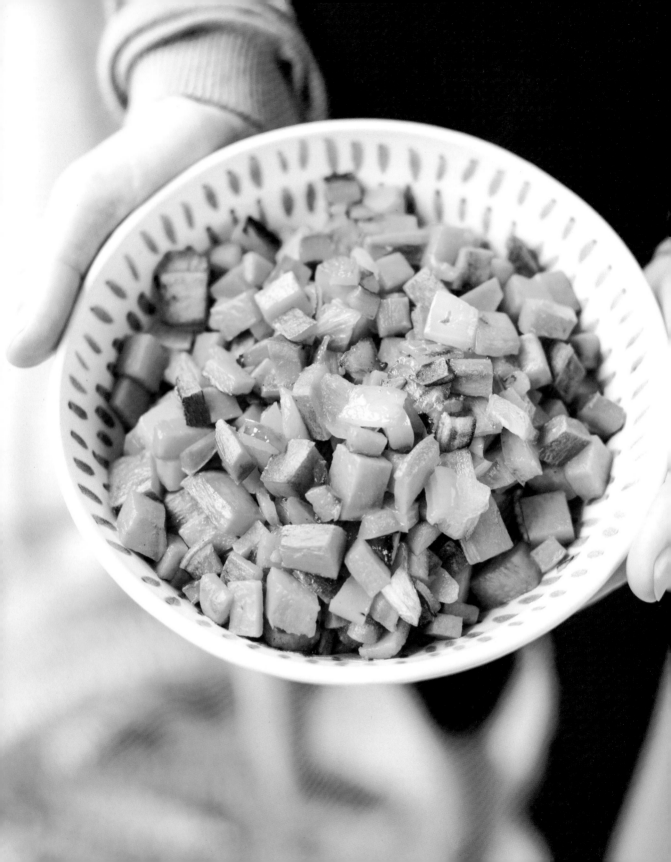

YAM HASH

I could eat this for every meal. It's quite possibly my favorite dish. You can also make it with red potatoes if you want to change it up. I choose yams over sweet potatoes because of the amazing hormone-balancing benefits and beta carotene. This recipe pairs well with the Socca Pancake on page 141.

Makes 4 Servings

2 large yams
½ red onion, diced
1 red or green bell pepper, seeded and diced
1 teaspoon jalapeño, minced (optional)
2–3 tablespoons coconut oil
1 teaspoon pink salt
1 teaspoon black pepper

Wash yams, cutting out any buried spots. Leave the skin on for this recipe. Dice into ¼-inch pieces. Set aside.

Preheat iron skillet on your stove top with oil in it. Once the skillet is hot, add in onion, bell pepper, and jalapeño if using. Cook for 10 minutes on medium, until onions are golden brown.

Toss in the yams, salt, and black pepper. You may need to add a little more coconut oil depending on how the potatoes soak it up.

Cook for 30 minutes until soft but crispy! Eat alone or as an amazing side dish.

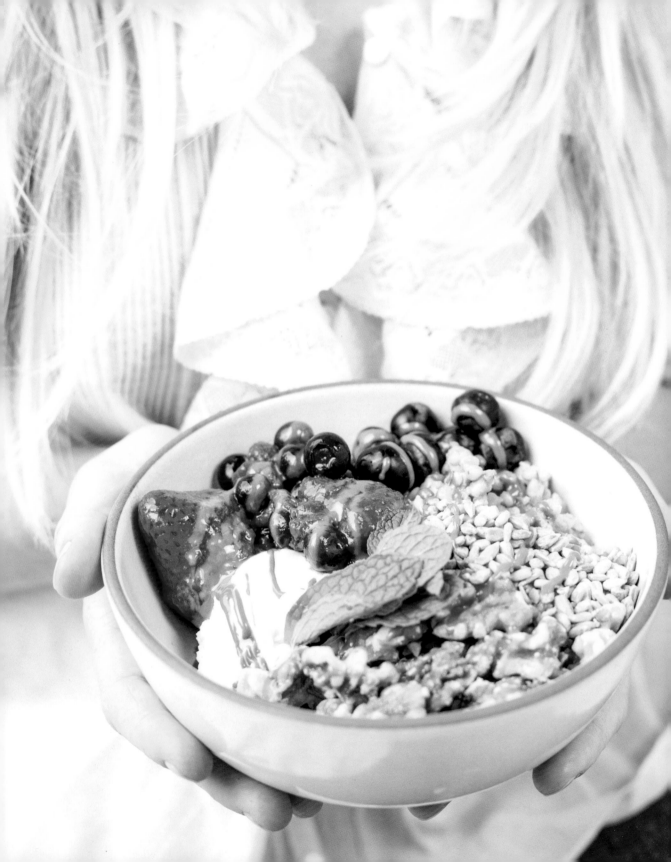

BUCKWHEAT PORRIDGE

This buckwheat recipe is made just like you would make oatmeal. Buckwheat is my son Henry's second-favorite breakfast (the Protein Pancakes on page 137 rank #1). I like that this porridge can be either savory or sweet depending on what you're in the mood for. If you enjoy butter (I do!) then adding some high-quality raw butter to this recipe gives it a little extra depth. You can top with whatever seasonal fruit delights you as well as any nuts, seeds, and butters.

Makes 2 Servings

base
1½ cups buckwheat groats
2½ cups water
½ teaspoon pink salt
1 tablespoon coconut oil
1 tablespoon raw butter (optional)
2 tablespoons raw honey or maple syrup, or favorite sweetener

toppings
Walnuts
Berries
Coconut yogurt
Sunflower seeds
Mint
Almond butter

In a medium saucepan pour in buckwheat, water, salt, and coconut oil and bring to a boil. Let cook for 5 minutes and then reduce to medium heat and cover with a lid for 30 minutes, stirring occasionally.

Once buckwheat is done, transfer to a bowl and add butter if using, and sweetener of choice.

Top with your favorite fruit and superfoods.

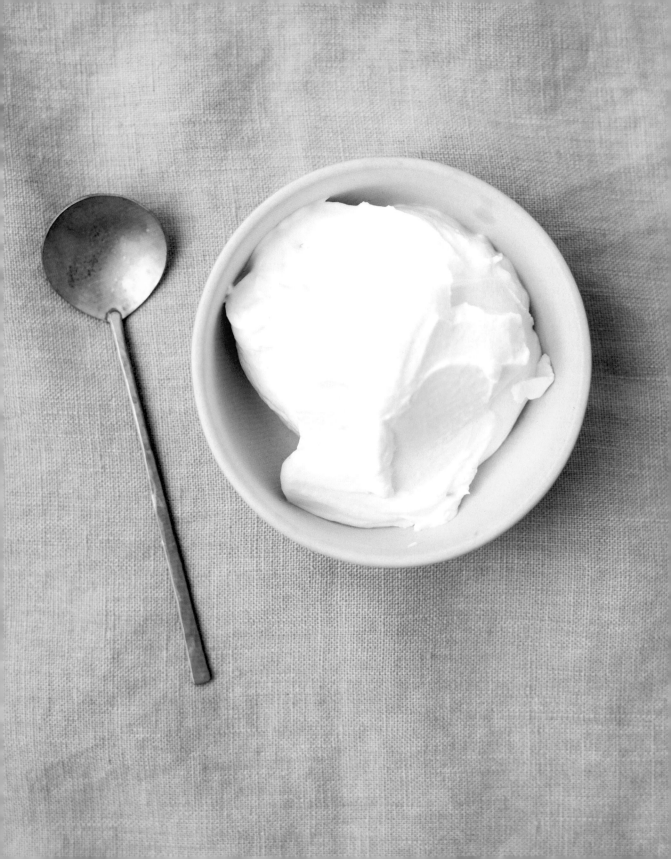

COCONUT YOGURT

It's light, creamy, and full of healthy, active, gut-loving probiotics. It's the ultimate beauty food. I love adding a bit to my chia pudding, or creating parfaits as pictured. So much beauty in nature's gifts. If you don't have access to young coconut, that's okay. Use one can of coconut milk (liquid drained) instead of the coconut flesh. This yogurt pairs perfectly with the Turmeric + Pepita Granola on page 151. In this recipe I use coconut milk powder—my favorite brand is Anima Mundi, which can be found online. We also sell it at Local Juicery if you happen to be in Sedona! I love it so much I actually eat it out of the bag. It's that good.

Makes 2 Cups

---

2 cups young coconut meat
  (about three coconuts)
2 cups coconut milk powder
Just a bit of coconut water for
  blending
2 teaspoons vegan powdered
  probiotic

NOTE: I love this yogurt topped with berries, granola, fresh fruit, bananas, nuts, and seeds

Remove coconut flesh from the young coconut and place in a high-speed blender.

Add the powdered coconut and a little water for blending, no more than ¼ cup.

Blend on high until very creamy, then add in the probiotic and blend quickly to combine.

Move to a glass bowl—it is important that the mixture is placed in a glass bowl, as metal will affect the fermentation process—and set in a warm dark area with a cloth over top for 2 to 3 days and then put it in a sealable glass jar.

Keeps the refrigerator for up to 1 month

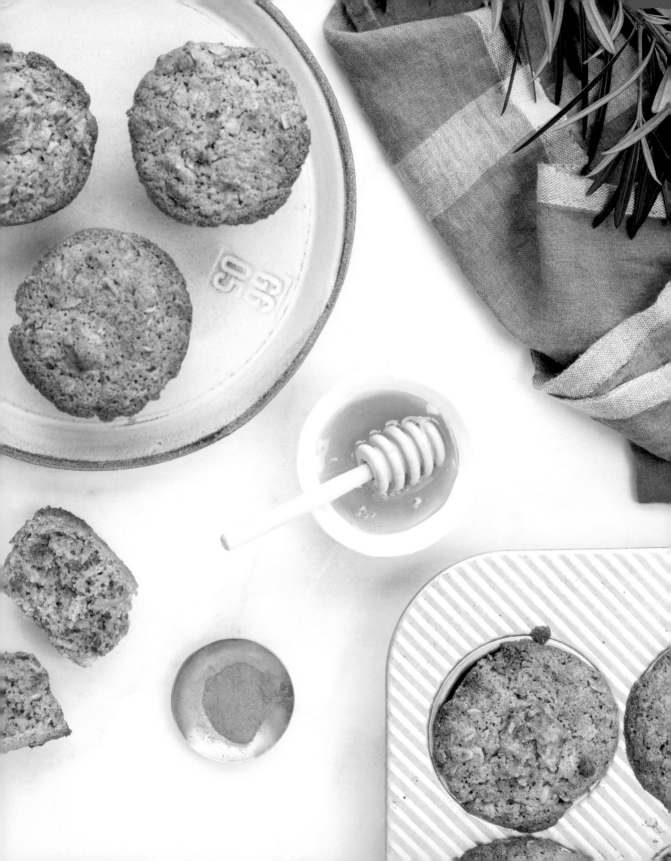

CARROT WALNUT RAISIN MUFFINS

I love dessert—anytime I can make breakfast more like dessert, I do. I love how filled with goodness these muffins are. They remind me of Grandma's muffins, but way healthier. I love keeping these in the fridge and then toasting them up and slathering on some raw grass-fed butter or coconut oil for a quick and nutritious breakfast.

Makes 16 Muffins

---

1 cup gluten-free oats
1½ cups almond flour
¼ cup arrowroot
¼ cup rice or millet flour
½ cup coconut sugar
¼ teaspoon baking soda
¾ teaspoon baking powder
1 cup crushed walnuts
⅓ cup raisins
½ teaspoon nutmeg
2 tablespoons cinnamon
½ teaspoon salt
6 carrots
3 eggs
¾ cup maple syrup
½ cup coconut oil, melted
2 tablespoons vanilla extract
1 teaspoon apple cider vinegar

Preheat oven to 350°F.

In metal bowl, combine oats, almond flour, arrowroot, rice flour, coconut sugar, baking soda, and baking powder, walnuts, raisins, nutmeg, cinnamon, and salt. Stir well and set aside.

Place the shredding blade on your food processor and shred the carrots. To the carrots, add eggs, maple syrup, melted coconut oil, vanilla, and apple cider vinegar. Use a whisk to combine.

Pour the wet mix into the dry mix and stir until well combined.

Line a muffin pan with muffin cups and fill to the brim of the paper. Cook for 35 minutes or until golden brown and soft in the middle.

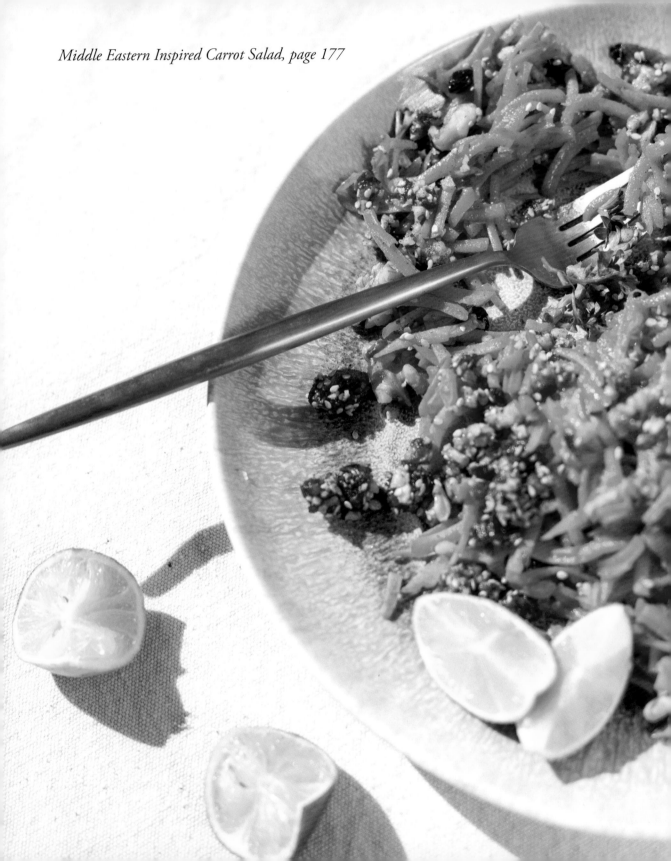

Middle Eastern Inspired Carrot Salad, page 177

SALADS

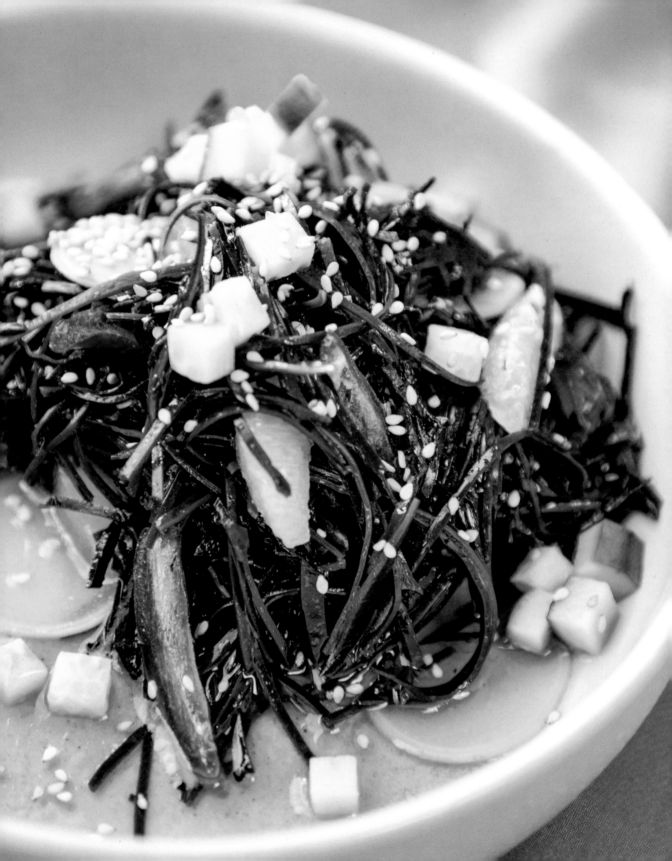

SIMPLE SEAWEED SALAD

I get really intense cravings for this seaweed salad! I first discovered it at a little co-op in Belfast, Maine. I couldn't get enough. This is my attempt to re-create a classic.

Makes 4 Servings

---

salad

1 cup dry seaweed of choice (I love arame)
1 cup Persian cucumbers, chopped
2 oranges, segmented
3 red radishes, thinly sliced
2 dates, pitted and sliced
Sesame seeds (optional)

dressing

2 teaspoons orange zest
½ cup orange juice, fresh
2 tablespoons rice vinegar
2 tablespoons Nama Shoyu
½ teaspoon sesame oil
1 tablespoon olive oil

Soak seaweed in water for about 10 minutes while you prepare the dressing and toppings.

make the dressing: In a medium bowl, combine all dressing ingredients and whisk until well combined.

assemble the salad: In a medium bowl, toss strained seaweed, cucumbers, segmented orange, radish slices, and dates with the dressing. With tongs, place the seaweed mixture into a bowl, then pour the remaining dressing in. Top with sesame seeds if desired.

NOTE: This salad is wonderful on a bed of spring greens if you would like more texture.

PISTACHIO + BEET CARPACCIO SALAD

The colors of this simple salad are beautiful. I love how the beets and the fennel go together so well, and the macadamia nut cheese and pistachios give it a richness that will keep you full and energized.

Makes 2 Servings

---

2 beets
2 tablespoons extra-virgin olive oil
1 fennel bulb, shaved
½ cup pistachios, crushed
Thick balsamic vinegar for drizzling
Black pepper to taste
Pink salt to taste
¼ cup macadamia nut cheese (page 261)

NOTE: For slicing thin veggies, use a mandoline for best results.

Using a mandoline or very sharp knife, thinly slice the beets. Put into a large bowl and toss with just a bit of olive oil and a pinch of salt.

Rinse the mandoline and slice the fennel thinly. Arrange beets and fennel on plates and then toss pistachios over top.

Drizzle balsamic vinegar, cracked pepper, and salt to taste. Top with crumbles of macadamia nut cheese.

MASTER KALE SALAD

Nothing makes me happier than an awesome, well-massaged and marinated kale salad, and nothing makes me more sad than a poorly executed one. I think if everyone experienced a well-massaged and marinated kale salad, the world would be a healthier place! If you're not marinating and massaging your kale, get ready for a next-level hack that will change your salad life from here on out. I like a little sweet in my salads, and this particular salad always feels great to my digestion. You just have to start to watch your body and how it responds to different combinations and you'll get your own flow going.

Makes 4 Servings

2 heads dinosaur kale, stems removed, thinly chopped
1 lemon, juiced
½ teaspoon pink salt
2 tablespoons extra-virgin olive oil
1 avocado, chopped
1 red bell pepper, seeded and diced
1 small apple, diced
½ cup hemp seeds
½ cup walnuts, lightly toasted and crushed
1 cup roasted or sautéed yam or butternut squash
3 dates, pitted and chopped
1 fennel bulb, thinly sliced

Place all the prepped kale in a large bowl and add lemon, pink salt, and olive oil. Massage the kale with your hands until each leaf is saturated.

Add in avocado, bell pepper, apple, hemp seeds, walnuts, yam or squash, dates, and fennel, toss gently, and then plate and enjoy.

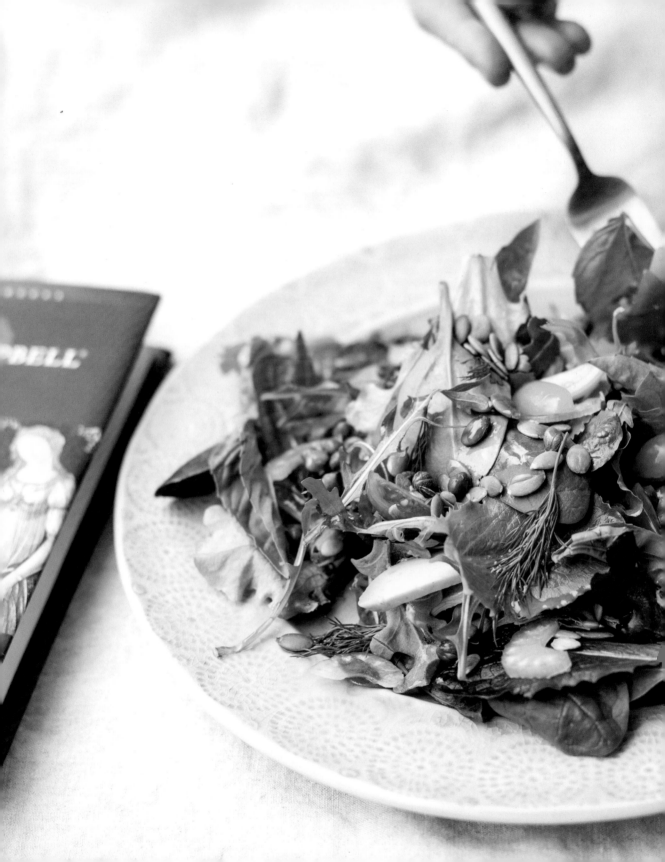

MY GO-TO SALAD

This is my typical to-go salad. I add it all into a nice glass storage bowl. I like to keep all the ingredients separate so they don't get soggy. The olive oil and lemon I put into another little side dish to they don't wilt the lettuce. Once you ready to eat you just pour in the dressing and shake! Perfect for traveling days or when you're going from meeting to meeting! I love the herbs, and the capers give a unique texture and flavor. Great for a wonderful side dinner salad or even for a main meal. I sometimes add some baked yam and cashew "Ricotta" from page 265 to make it more filling and round out the nutrients.

Makes 2 Servings

1 head green leaf lettuce, chopped
1 cup arugula
2 celery stalks, sliced
1 small avocado, diced
10 baby tomatoes, quartered
½ cup cilantro, minced
¼ cup basil, minced
¼ cup dill, minced
2 tablespoons capers
¼ cup pumpkin seeds
Extra-virgin olive oil, lemon, pink salt, and black pepper to taste

In a large bowl combine lettuce, arugula, celery, avocado, tomatoes, cilantro, basil, dill, capers, and pumpkin seeds.

Add olive oil, lemon, salt, and black pepper to taste.

Toss and enjoy!

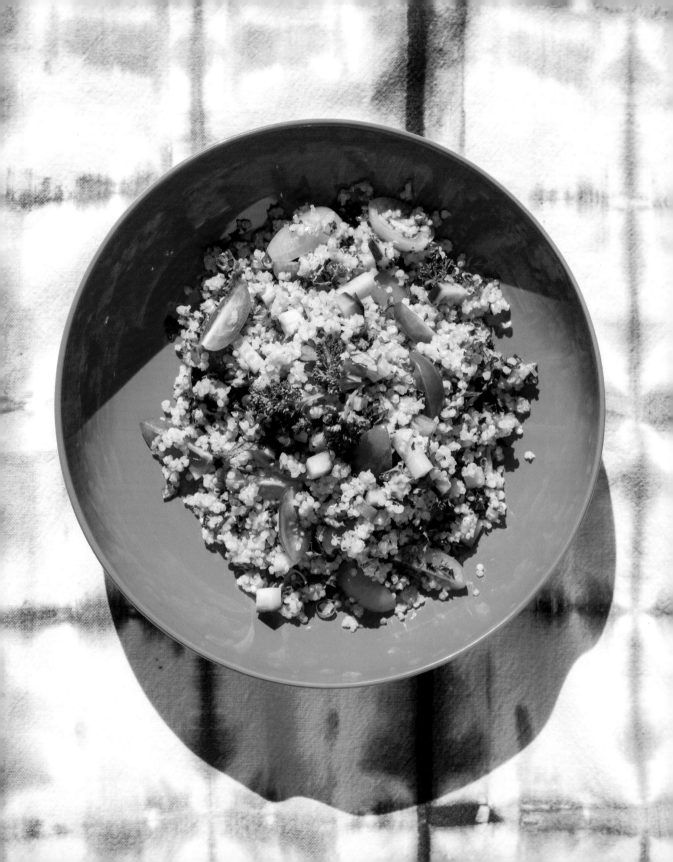

QUINOA TABBOULEH SALAD

I love traditional Lebanese tabbouleh, but I don't often eat wheat (though indulging in traditionally made tabbouleh with bulgur wheat once in a great while is still something I do). Quinoa offers a great high-protein alternative to the wheat. The sweet tomatoes and fresh herbs are so refreshing. I think you'll love this as much as I do!

Makes 6 Servings

---

1 small garlic clove, minced

2 cucumbers, peeled and very finely chopped

1 cup fresh parsley, minced

½ cup mint, minced

½ pound ripe tomatoes, very finely chopped

4 scallions, finely chopped

1 cup cooked quinoa, cooled

2–3 lemons, juiced (to taste)

¼ cup extra-virgin olive oil

Salt, to taste

In a bowl combine garlic, cucumbers, parsley, mint, tomatoes, and scallions.

Add vegetables into the cooled quinoa. Add in the lemon juice, olive oil, and salt to taste.

Toss and enjoy!

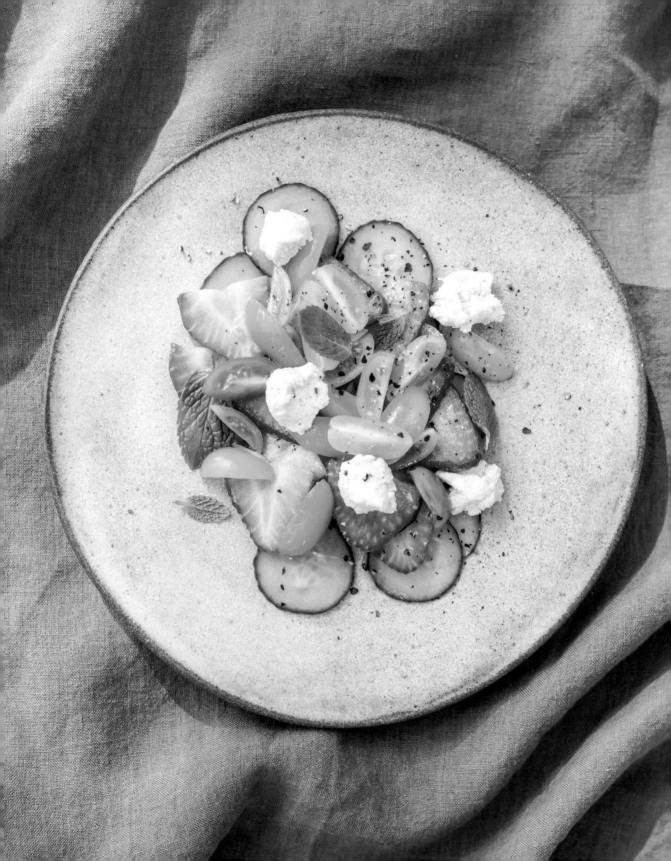

SUMMERTIME SALAD

This is such a delight to look at. It's a joy to eat also. The perfect combination of sweet, tart, and crisp. I use just a light dressing that's lemon-based, which brings out the flavor even more. This is the perfect salad for an outdoor midsummer dinner.

Makes 2 Servings

salad

1 cup baby tomatoes, quartered
1 cup strawberries, sliced thin
2 cucumbers, peeled and
  seeded
1 small bunch fresh mint
⅓ cup cashew "Ricotta" (page
  265) or macadamia nut butter
  (page 261)
Salt and pepper to taste

dressing

⅓ cup lime or lemon juice
1½ tablespoons raw honey
⅓ cup extra-virgin olive oil
¼ teaspoon garlic powder
  (optional)
Salt and pepper

make the salad: In a bowl, lightly toss tomatoes, strawberries, and cucumbers in dressing. Then place delicately on a plate, arranging so that all the colors show.

Top with fresh mint, ricotta, and salt and cracked pepper.

make the dressing: In a bowl, whisk together all ingredients until well blended.

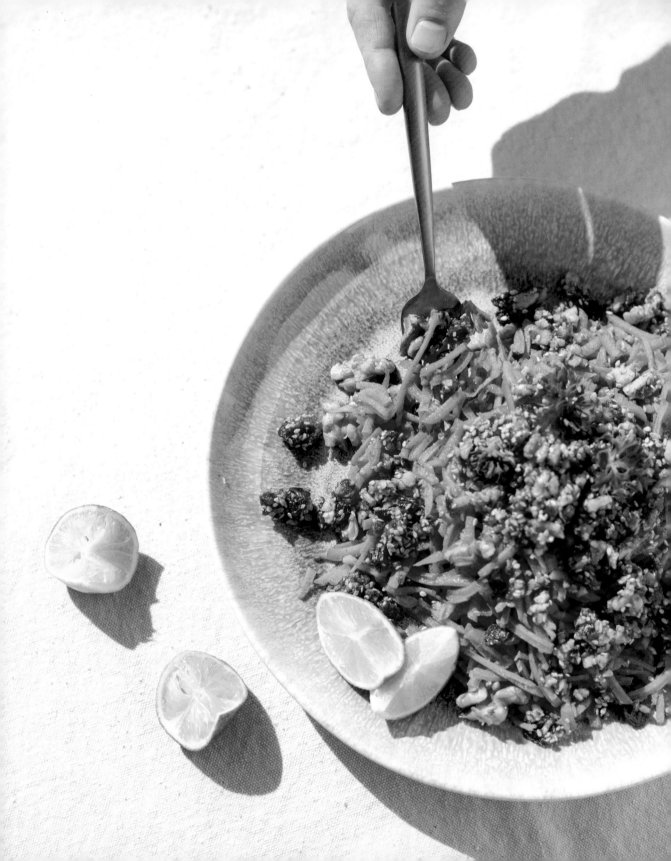

MIDDLE-EASTERN-INSPIRED CARROT SALAD

Carrots are such loves! So versatile, you can eat them in so many ways and in so many dishes, but this is one of my favorite ways to enjoy these sweet roots. Sweet, crunchy, spiced, and with just the right amount of tartness, this salad is perfect for a warm summer day or as a side dish to a large meal.

Makes 2 Servings

---

salad
5 cups carrots, shredded
1 cup walnuts, toasted
½ cup raisins or goji berries
1 cup dukkah (page 206)

dressing
4 tablespoons extra-virgin olive
 oil
1 teaspoon cinnamon
¼ teaspoon cumin
2 lemons, squeezed
½ teaspoon salt

make the dressing: Whisk together olive oil, cinnamon, cumin, lemon juice, and salt.

make the salad: Place carrots in a large mixing bowl. Add in toasted walnuts, raisins, and dressing. Toss until all carrots are covered with dressing. Plate and then top with the dukkah.

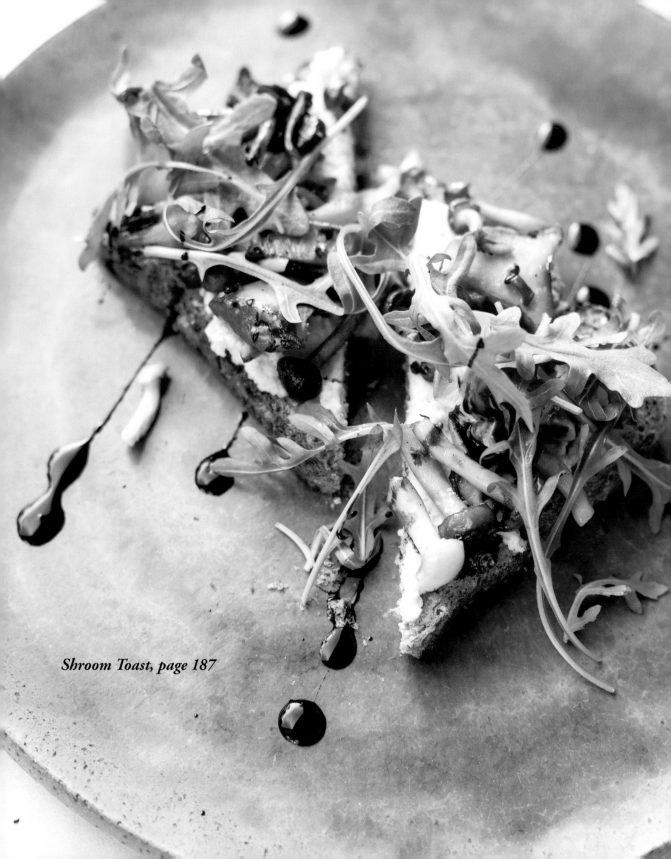

Shroom Toast, page 187

SANDWICHES, WRAPS + TOASTS

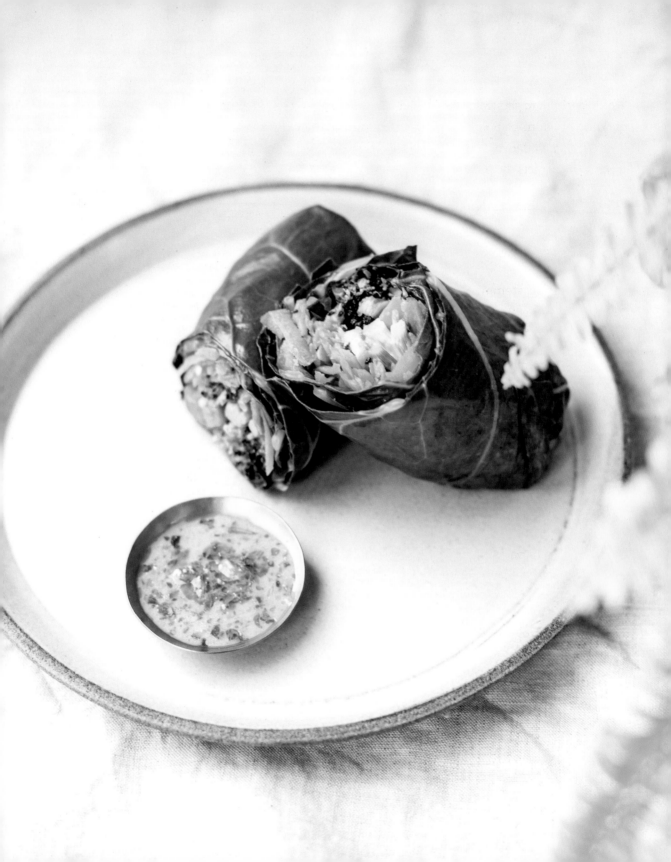

THE WRAP WRAP

Wraps like this are perfect for next-day lunches. I make them ahead of time and take them with me; they save me from grabbing something that I won't be proud of later in the day. You can fill them with whatever you love! This is my personal favorite—the chimichurri is delicious, and the protein for the tempeh gets me thought that three o'clock slump.
Makes 4 Wraps

---

sauce
1 bunch fresh cilantro, stemmed and chopped
½ bunch parsley, stemmed and chopped
1 teaspoon oregano
½ teaspoon garlic powder
½ small shallot, minced
½ cup extra-virgin olive oil
2 tablespoon lemon juice
½ teaspoon pink salt

filling
½ shallot, minced
1–2 tablespoons coconut oil
2 cups roasted or steamed broccoli heads
1 cup Yam Hash (page 157)
Pink salt to taste

wrap
4–6 pieces of nori, quickly steamed collards, or your favorite tortilla—whatever you choose works great
2 tablespoons Macadamia Nut Butter (page 261), or almond butter

make the sauce: In a small bowl combine all sauce ingredients and whisk with a fork until blended. Set aside.

make the filling: In a small frying pan, sauté the shallot in coconut oil and add in the broccoli (if using steamed; you don't need to sauté broccoli if you are using roasted).

Cook for 3 to 5 minutes until onions are golden. Add in the yam hash for 1 minute to warm and salt to taste.

assemble: Choose your wrap (I love the collards as pictured) and lay out flat on a cutting board. Spread the macadamia nut butter or almond butter on the side facing you.

Depending on your wrap size, add about ½ cup of the filling and then top with 2 tablespoons of the chimichurri sauce.

Salt if needed. Wrap and roll!

If you're saving these for another day, wrap in wax paper and tape closed.

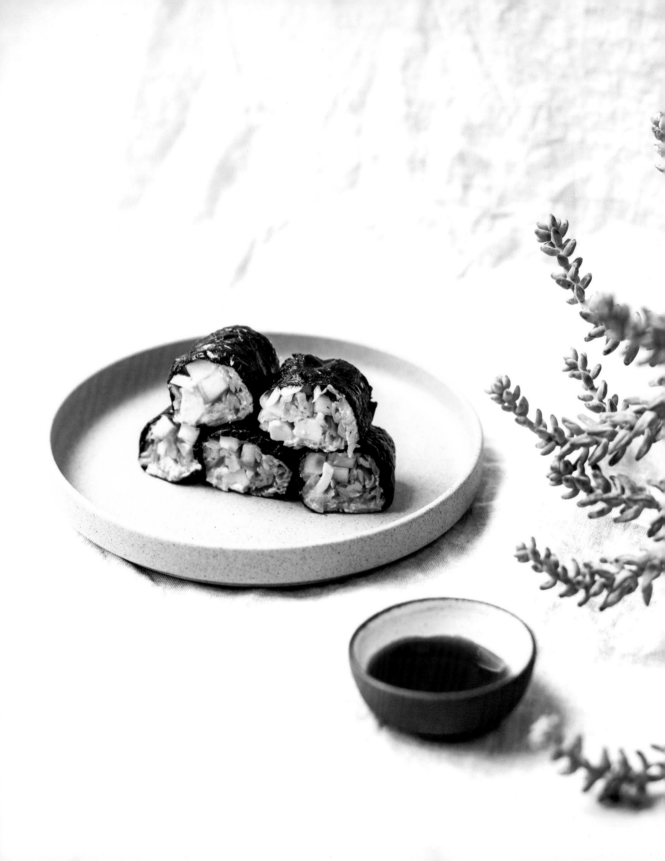

VEGETABLE + HUMMUS WRAP

Such a simple and easy lunch. Perfect for days when you just don't feel like being traditional. I love using nori that is traditionally used for sushi, which makes a perfect iodine-rich wrap. Collards and lettuce are great options too. You can get really playful with this kind of recipe, add in your favorite veggies, even a precooked and cooled grain if you desire. So many fun things to wrap.

Makes 2 Servings

2 nori, collards, or lettuce leaves
¼ cup Raffi's Hummus (page 259)
1 tablespoon almond butter
2 carrots, shredded or sliced
½ avocado, pit removed
4 tablespoons kimchi or
   sauerkraut
½ cucumber, peeled and sliced

Lay out your wrap of choice.

Spread the hummus and almond butter all over each wrap, then add the veggies to one side (think of wrapping a burrito or sushi).

Simply roll up and enjoy!

MACADAMIA NUT RICOTTA + FIG CROSTINI

I adore fresh figs—the fruit, the tree, and the aroma. I also love the nutritional offerings: fiber, cleansing of mucus, and high iron! The macadamia nut ricotta is creamy and delicious and the hint of sweet from the fig is the perfect touch. Great for dinner parties or a decadent lunch.

Makes 6 Toasts

6 slices Simple Seed Bread
   (page 257)
1 cup macadamia nut butter
   (page 261)
6 fresh figs, sliced
4 tablespoons hazelnuts, toasted
Extra-virgin olive oil for drizzling
Wildflower honey for drizzling
Syrupy balsamic vinegar, for
   drizzling
Zest of ½ Meyer lemon

Toast Simple Seed Bread until golden brown and then spread macadamia nut butter on each slice.

Layer with fresh figs, hazelnuts, olive oil, honey, vinegar, and then top with zest.

Plate and enjoy!

NOTE: If figs aren't in season, you can use pear or any other favorite fruit. I love peaches for this as well.

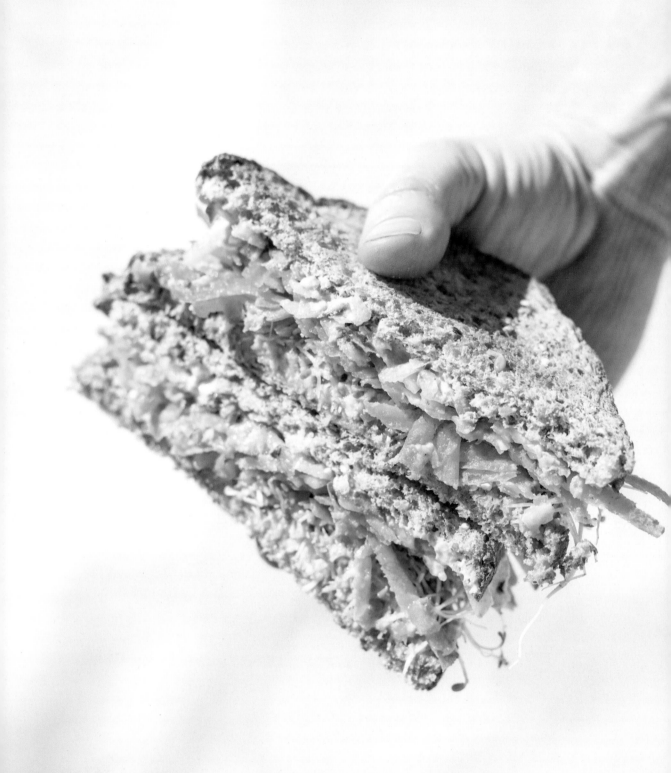

CLASSIC VEGGIE SANDWICH

When I was a kid, this was my favorite go-to sandwich, and I still crave it! I find that the Vegenaise really brings the flavor together, but you're welcome to replace it with Cashew Cheese (page 261) or whatever creamy spread you love!

Makes 1 Sandwich

2 slices sprouted grain bread
1 tablespoon Vegenaise
¼ large avocado
1 tablespoon hummus
Pink salt to taste
Small handful of fresh sprouts
¼ cup carrots, shredded
¼ cup cucumber, shredded
1 lettuce leaf

Toast the bread until it's light golden brown. Spread Vegenaise on one side of each slice of toasted bread.

Mash avocado and hummus into both sides and sprinkle with some salt.

Add the sprouts, shredded veggies, and lettuce to one side of the sandwich and then top with your remaining piece of bread. Slice and enjoy!

LUNCH ON THE GO, GO

This is one of the easiest grab-and-go lunches. It's a simple wrap with great nutrition. You can use whatever you have and make it a meal. My staples are greens, nut butter, and sauerkraut. If I have leftover rice or quinoa, I'll toss that in, too.

Makes 2 Servings

2 nori sheets
2 handfuls fresh or steamed greens
2 large scoops sauerkraut
1 tablespoon nut or seed butter
1 carrot, thinly sliced
¼ cucumber, thinly sliced
Small handful Greek olives, sliced or whole
¼ avocado, thinly sliced
2 tablespoons coconut aminos for dipping, optional

Lay out the nori sheets. Layer in ingredients on one side the nori, starting with the greens, sauerkraut, and nut butter.

Lay the carrot, cucumber, olives, and avocado on top.

Roll, starting with the side where the ingredients are stacked. Slowly fold and continue to roll. Dip in coconut aminos if desired.

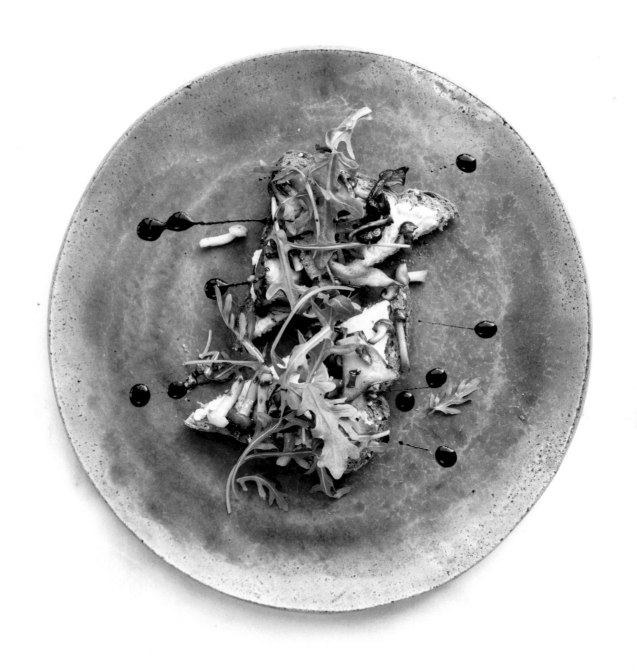

SHROOM TOAST

This recipe is out-of-this-world delicious. I use the Simple Seed Bread from page 257, but it's also delicious on a rustic sourdough or sprouted grain. The mushrooms cook in coconut oil and seasoning, and they really soak in all the flavors. It's a very comforting and unique meal. I like it with microgreens and a little Cashew Cheese spread on the bread (page 261), you could even add a little bit of fig compote or chutney.

Makes 4 Toasts

---

mushrooms
4 cups favorite mushrooms, thinly sliced
½ teaspoon maple syrup
½ teaspoon pink salt
½ teaspoon black pepper
4 tablespoon coconut oil or pastured butter

toast + toppings
4 slices favorite bread
½ cup macadamia nut butter (page 261)
1 cup arugula
Thick vinegar for drizzling
Salt and pepper to taste

Place your sliced mushrooms in a bowl and add the maple syrup, salt, and pepper.

Heat up skillet with coconut oil and add in mushroom mixture. Cook for 25 minutes until golden brown.

Once the mushrooms are finished, toast bread, spread on macadamia nut butter, place mushrooms and arugula on top, and drizzle with vinegar. Add salt and pepper to taste.

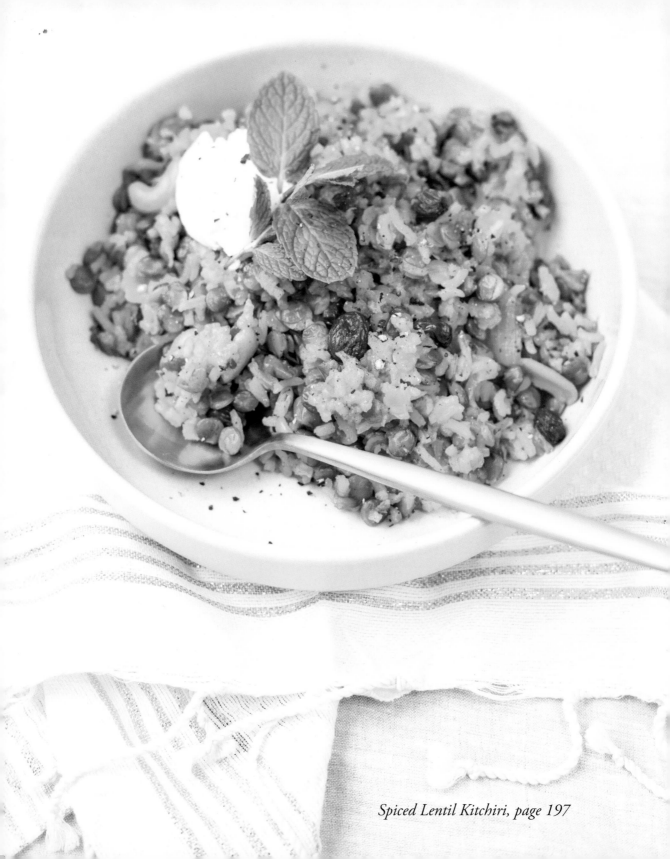

Spiced Lentil Kitchiri, page 197

SOUPS

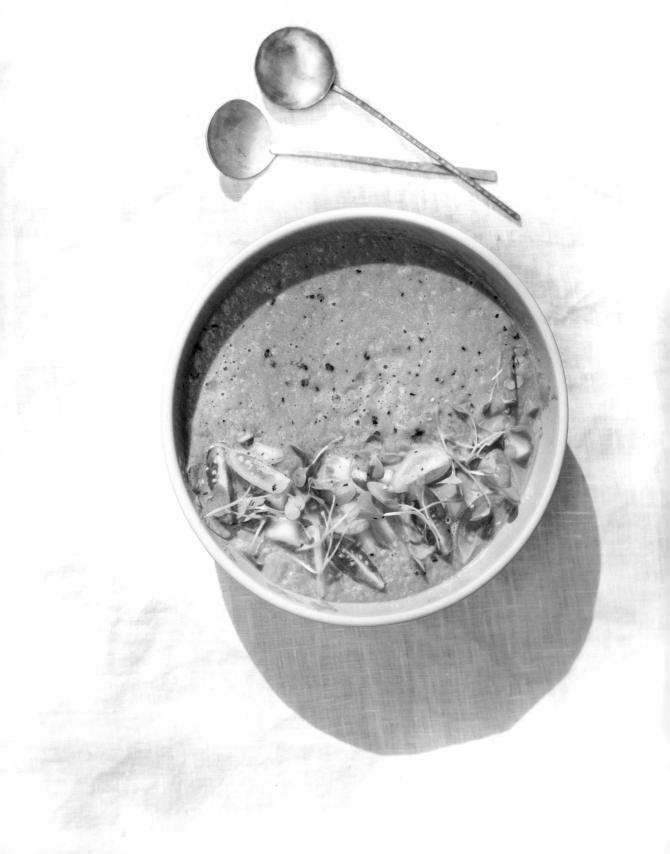

RAW SALAD SOUP

Clean, green, and really refreshing. The perfect simple lunch on a hot day. This is a classic raw food meal. I like the bit of sweetness from the carrots, the creaminess from the avocado and tahini, and the hydration from the spinach and cucumber. It's surprisingly filling and fun to eat. I sometimes spiralize some cucumber noodles and add them in for a fun texture.

Makes 2 Servings

1 cucumber, quartered
2 carrots, chopped
1 small jalapeño (optional)
2 cups spinach, tightly packed
½ avocado, pit removed
½–1 lemon, juiced
1 tablespoon tahini
½ teaspoon pink salt
½ cup water

Wash all vegetables and greens, then place them into a blender with the avocado.

Add in lemon juice, tahini, salt, and water.

Blend on high until creamy. Pour into your favorite bowl and enjoy!

SUMMER GAZPACHO

This is great for calming down on hot summer days. Lovely for dinner parties, it looks and tastes like it takes a lot of time, but really just takes minutes!

Makes 2 Servings

4 tomatoes, seeded and
  chopped
2 cups watermelon, no rind,
  chopped
½ cup basil, tightly packed
2 limes, juiced
1 tablespoon extra-virgin olive
  oil
½ teaspoon pink salt

Add tomatoes, chopped watermelon, basil, lime juice, olive oil, and pink salt to your blender or food processor.

Pulse until a salsa consistency forms. Don't over blend! This dish should be chunky.

Pour into a lovely glass bowl or cup and top with extra basil. Enjoy!

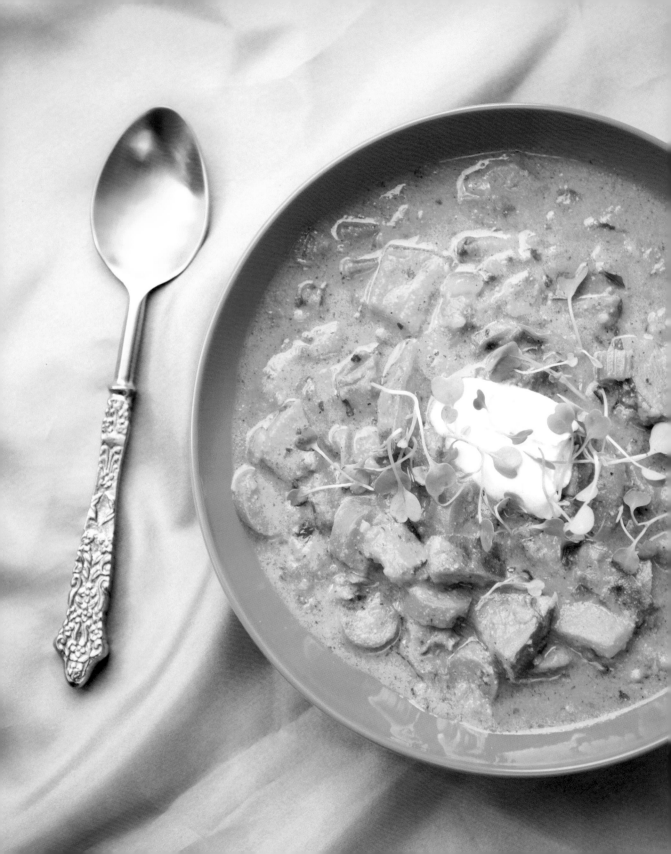

CLASSIC CURRY STEW

This is a great stew for the colder months of the year. It's wonderful for fighting any inflammation in the body and boosting the immune system. This is a perfect recipe for when the cold or flu is going around. If you aren't opposed to bone broth, you can use it as the base instead of water, which will support the immune system even more—making it a total wellness food. *Makes 12 Servings*

---

cashew cream
2 cup cashews
6 cups water

stew
4 cups carrots, diced
1 cup celery, sliced
1 cup onion, diced
¼ cup mint, minced
1 bunch cilantro, minced
1 cup basil, minced
½ cup jalapeño, minced
1 large thumb ginger, peeled
    and minced
1 cup coconut oil
8 yams, peeled and diced
1 tablespoon onion powder
2 tablespoons curry powder
¼ cup fresh turmeric, minced
3 cloves garlic, minced
1 tablespoon cumin
2 teaspoons cinnamon
1 teaspoon nutmeg
⅓ cup coconut sugar
¼ cup apple cider vinegar
6 cups cashew milk (page 101)
3 tablespoons salt
1 teaspoon black pepper
7 cups water

make the cashew cream: Blend 1 cup cashews with 3 cups of water two times (until you have roughly six cups). You don't need to strain this milk! Set aside after it's made.

make the stew: In the bottom of your soup pot, sauté carrots, celery, onion, mint, cilantro, basil, jalapeño, and ginger in coconut oil for 5 to 10 minutes. The onion should be translucent.

Add in diced yams, onion powder, curry powder, fresh turmeric, garlic, cumin, cinnamon, nutmeg, coconut sugar, and vinegar. Let cook a bit more and then add in the cashew milk, salt, black pepper, and water.

Cook for 35 minutes until it boils and then put on low and simmer for another 15 minutes.

> **NOTE:** This soup just gets better with time. Best served the day after once all the flavors have set in.

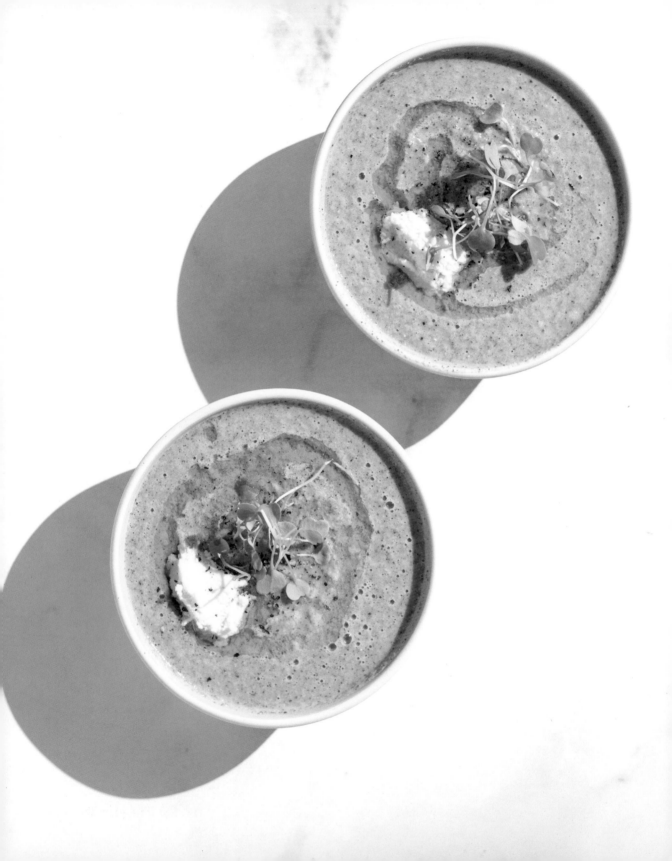

CREAM OF BROCCOLI SOUP

Another pregnancy favorite. I love this because you get all the benefits of broccoli but with the taste of cream. A win-win. Even my six-year-old loves this soup!

Makes 4 Servings

---

1 shallot, minced
2 tablespoons coconut oil, divided
2 heads broccoli, chopped
2 cups bone or vegetable broth
2 cups water
1 (12 ounce) can coconut cream
1 teaspoon onion powder
2 teaspoons salt

Sauté the shallot in a soup pan with 1 tablespoon of coconut oil until golden brown.

Add chopped broccoli to the shallot. Add in broth and water and bring broth to a boil.

Fill your blender halfway with broccoli and liquid and then add coconut cream, onion powder, salt, and remaining coconut oil. Blend until creamy.

Set aside and repeat the process until fully blended.

Pour into your favorite bowl and enjoy!

NOTE: Can be enjoyed hot or cold! Goes great with the Macadamia Nut Butter from page 261.

CHICKEN NOODLE SOUP

I don't prepare many animal products for my family, but whenever anyone gets a cold I do make this. I roast a local, pasture-raised chicken the night before so I have the bones for the broth and the meat for the soup. After roasting the chicken, I put the bones in the slow cooker and let them cook all night and make a really nourishing, medicinal broth. That's what makes this soup extra nourishing and special. If you're vegan you can make this with vegetable broth (page 263) and just add extra veggies!

Makes 2 Servings

---

1 head celery, diced
8 carrots, chopped
1 onion or shallot, chopped
3 tablespoons coconut oil
3 tablespoons fresh parsley, minced
1 teaspoon fresh thyme, minced
1 teaspoon fresh marjoram, minced
4 red potatoes, diced
2 cups roasted chicken
1 teaspoon salt
1 teaspoon black pepper
8 cups chicken bone broth (for a vegan version see page 263)
3 cups rice noodles, precooked

In a large soup pot, sauté celery, carrots, onion, and coconut oil until onion is translucent.

Add in parsley, thyme, marjoram, potatoes, and roasted chicken. Sauté for 5 minutes.

Add in salt, black pepper, and broth. Bring to a boil and then turn to low for about 40 minutes.

Add in noodles and bring temperature up to medium high for 5 to 8 minutes.

Pour into your favorite bowl and enjoy!

SPICED LENTIL KITCHIRI

A staple in my home during the autumn and winter months. Warming, simple, and so delicious. This is one of those soups that just gets better with age. I love it around day two, when all the spices are integrated and the flavors pop! The toppings are fun too—the options are endless. I share my favorite below. (Pictured on page 188.)

Makes 6 Servings

---

stew

1 large sweet onion, chopped
1 tablespoon ginger, minced
1 tablespoon turmeric, minced
3 tablespoons ghee, butter or
   coconut oil
10 ounces sprouted lentils
½ cup white basmati rice
5½ cups water
1 teaspoon cumin
1½ teaspoons turmeric powder
1 teaspoon cinnamon
½ teaspoon garlic powder
½ teaspoon ginger powder
½ teaspoon coriander powder
½ lemon, juiced
1–2 tablespoons pink salt
¾ cup coconut milk
⅓ cup raisins
⅔ cup cashews

toppings
Lime
Cilantro
Cashew Crema (page 259)

In a medium saucepan, combine onion, ginger, and turmeric, and sauté in ghee or coconut oil for about 10 minutes.

Add in lentils and rice, and cook for about 5 minutes.

Add water, cumin, turmeric, cinnamon, garlic, ginger, coriander, lemon juice, salt, coconut milk, and raisins. Bring to a boil, then reduce heat to low, cover, and cook for 30 minutes, stirring occasionally.

Add in cashews and cook for 5 more minutes. Turn off heat and let cool.

Serve with fresh lime, cilantro, and cashew crema.

> **NOTE:** Pairs well with the Socca Pancake on page 141.

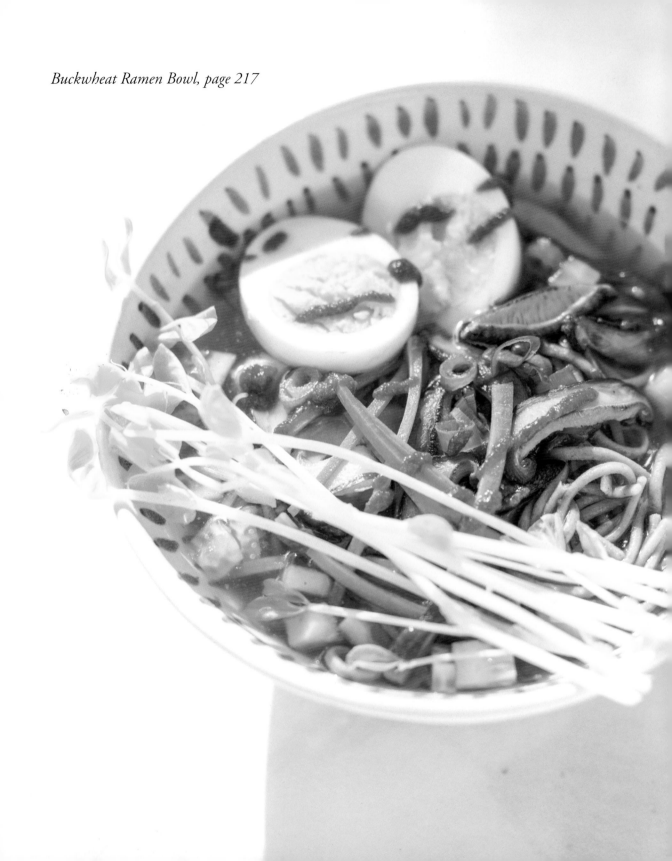

Buckwheat Ramen Bowl, page 217

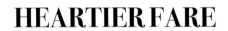

HEARTIER FARE

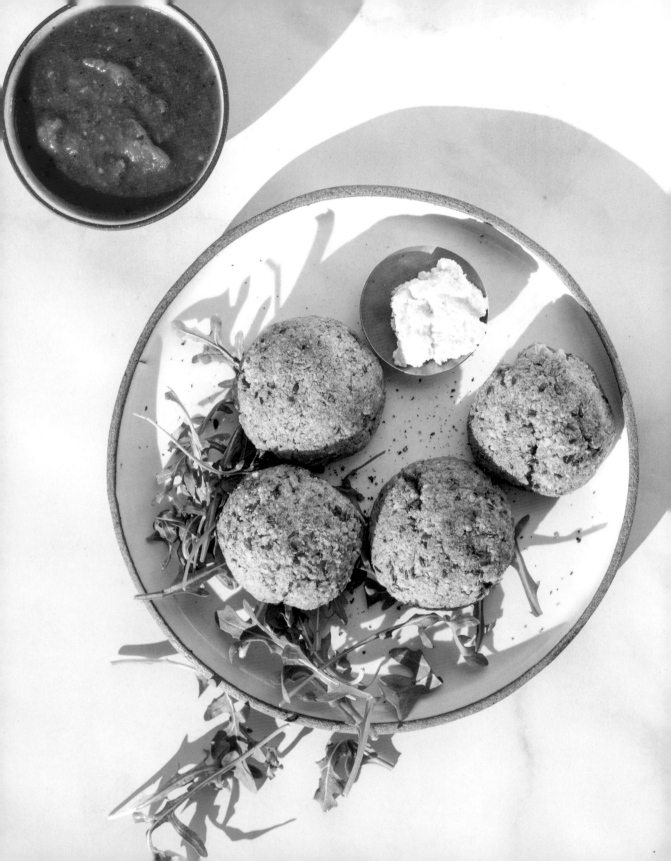

MARINARA + WALNUT "MEAT" BALLS

A dreamy meal, that's what this is. It's completely comforting and satisfying without being too heavy. I made this a lot during my pregnancy. I use zucchini noodles, but you can really use whatever noodle you love. The meatballs are made from lentils and walnuts, so they are filled with healthy protein, and the sauce has so many vegetables! If you're really wanting to indulge, add a little fresh Parmesan or goat cheese on top—it will tip it over the edge. For the tomatoes, I always buy tomato paste and crushed tomatoes in glass jars. I add in fresh baby ones as well.
Makes 4 Servings

---

meatballs
2 cups cooked lentils or rice (page 251)
2 cups walnuts
1 tablespoon ground flaxseed
1 tablespoon psyllium husk
2 tablespoons coconut oil
1½ tablespoons garlic
2 teaspoons shallot, minced
2 tablespoons fresh parsley, minced
1 teaspoon oregano
1 date, pitted
1 teaspoon salt

sauce
1 tablespoon extra-virgin olive oil
1 red onion, diced
1 cup fresh basil, minced
3 carrots, diced
2 cups fresh baby tomatoes, quartered
8 ounces tomato paste
1 (32 ounce) can crushed tomatoes
2 teaspoons pink salt
2 teaspoons apple cider vinegar

make the meatballs: Preheat oven to 375°F. In a food processor combine all meatball ingredients. Process until a crumbly cookie dough consistency forms. Roll into 2-inch balls and place on a parchment paper–lined baking sheet. Bake for 30 minutes on the middle rack. Should be a nice golden brown when finished. Leave on the pan to cool and then use a spatula to remove them from the pan.

make the sauce: Add olive oil to a large saucepan then add onion. Cook until onions are transparent. Add in basil, carrots, and baby tomatoes. Cook for 10 minutes, stirring occasionally. Add in tomato paste, crushed tomatoes, salt, and vinegar. Simmer for 30 to 40 minutes on low. Place meatballs on top of sauce after plating. These don't cook well in the sauce as traditional ones do.

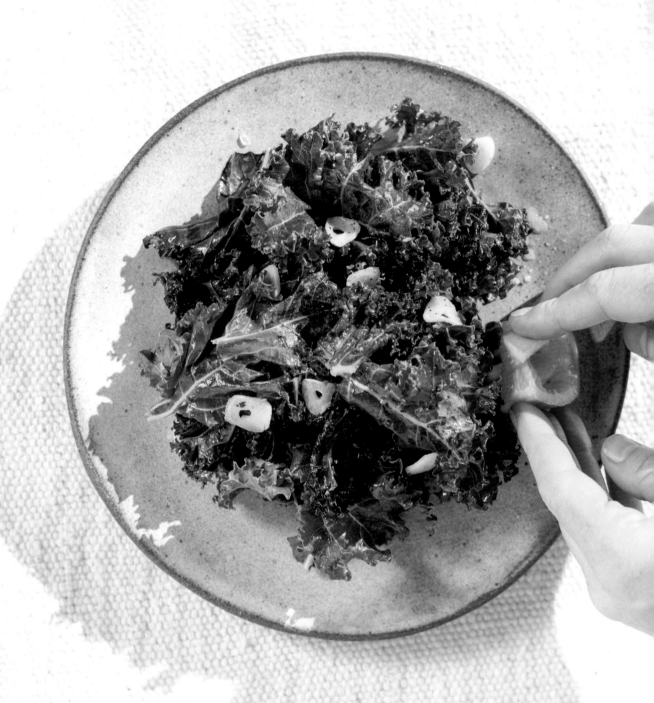

SAUTÉED DINNER GREENS

Restaurant style! These simple-to-make greens pull together any meal. I prep my greens a couple days ahead of time to make throwing a dish like this together even easier. Pairs well with a simple baked potato or even as a topping to any soup.

Makes 4 Servings

2 tablespoons coconut oil or
    extra-virgin olive oil
2 garlic cloves, sliced
½ shallot, minced
3 heads kale, chard, or collards,
    stems removed
½ teaspoon salt
Pepper to taste
Lemon to taste

In a large frying pan add oil, garlic, and shallots and cook for 5 minutes.

Add greens, salt, and pepper, and sauté for another 5 to 8 minutes.

Place on a large plate and squeeze lemon all over!

LEAN AND CLEAN LASAGNA

This is pretty much vegan comfort food; we all need it once in a while. This is a favorite in my house. My family always knows when I'm making it—it makes the house smell divine. I made this a lot though my pregnancy when I was craving heavier foods. This did the trick! Satisfying and still full of veggies.

Makes 6–8 Servings

2 packages gluten-free lasagna
    noodles
8 carrots, chopped
1 large yellow summer squash
6 kale leaves, stemmed
1 red onion, diced
1 pound spinach
1 tablespoon coconut oil
2 bottles of your favorite marinara
    sauce, or see page 201
2 cups Cashew
    Cheese (page 261)

Preheat oven to 380°F.

Cook lasagna noodles according to instructions.

Sauté carrots, squash, kale, red onion, and spinach in coconut oil until soft. Set aside.

In a casserole pan, start layering noodles: one layer on the bottom, then ¼ of the sauce, vegetables, and cashew cheese. Keep layering until all ingredients are gone! Top with marinara.

Bake for 45 minutes and then serve!

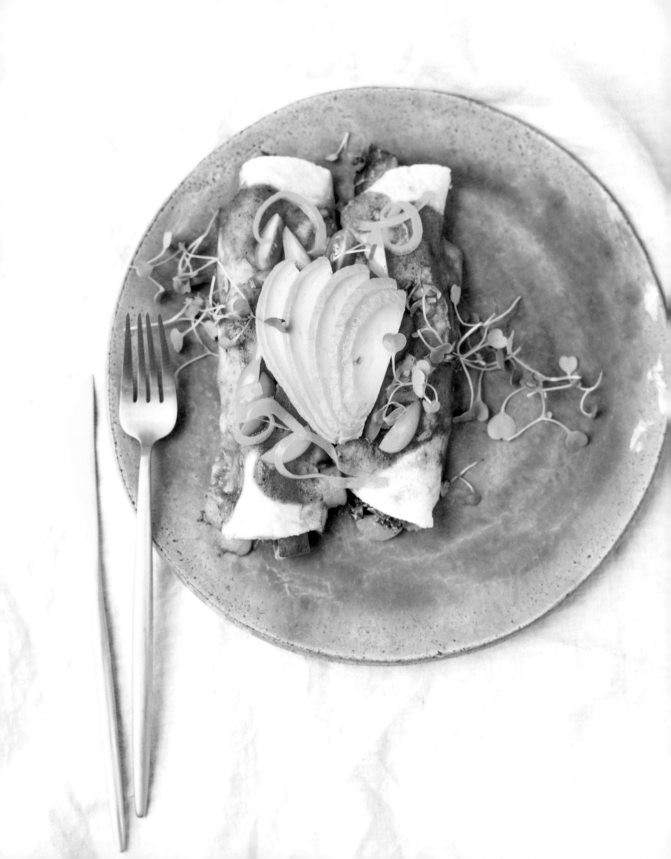

VEGETABLE ENCHILADAS

If you're still thinking that plant-based food is boring and flavorless, I think this recipe will finally turn you. You won't even miss traditional enchiladas, this recipe is so flavor filled and comforting while still packing a nutritious punch! I sometimes add in raw organic cheddar cheese if I'm feeling it! See note for amounts.

Makes 4 Servings

---

1 onion, chopped

2 yams, chopped

6 carrots, chopped

3 cups kale, stemmed and chopped

1 tablespoon coconut oil

Salt to taste

12 tortillas (I love Siete grain-free brand)

1 (16 ounce) can black beans, or recipe from page 267

2 cups brown rice (page 273)

2 cups red enchilada sauce (I buy a premade organic version)

Chilies or jalapeños

¼ cup black olives, sliced

Preheat oven to 350°F.

In a frying pan, sauté onion, yams, carrots, and kale in coconut oil until golden brown. Salt to taste. Set aside.

On a large cutting board, fill each tortilla with about ¼ cup vegetables and 3 tablespoons beans and rice, roll, and place into casserole dish. Continue until you are out of vegetables.

Pour enchilada sauce over the entire dish, then top with chilies or jalapeños and black olives. If you love cheese, add this on too!

Bake for 35 to 40 minutes.

Let cool for 5 to 10 minutes, then enjoy!

NOTE: I don't typically eat cheese, but if you love it, this would be the dish to add it to. Also goes great with cultured sour cream! I use about 2 cups of grated raw organic cheddar, I toss it right on top!

VEGETABLE CRUDITÉS WITH WALNUT DUKKAH + HUMMUS

The walnut dukkah and the hummus are both inspired by our dear friend Raffi. He's from Syria and always sharing his mother's recipes with our family. Besides sharing amazing recipes and always having open arms to us, they are the most giving and grateful family I've ever met. Not once have I ever heard a complaint from them—not once. I have so much respect for their warmth and positivity. This meal is perfect for sharing and enjoying on a warm spring day.
Makes 2 Servings

---

dukkah

1 cup walnuts, lightly toasted and crushed
½ cup sesame seeds, lightly toasted
½ cup dates, pitted and chopped
2 tablespoons coriander seeds
1 tablespoon cumin
1 teaspoon ground sumac
½ teaspoon pink salt
⅛ cup extra-virgin olive oil

assembly

5 heirloom carrots, sliced lengthwise
4 celery stalks, sliced lengthwise
1 cup baby tomatoes
2 cups lightly steamed cauliflower
6 lettuce leaves
Raffi's Hummus (page 259)

make the dukkah: In a food processor, combine all dukkah ingredients.

Pulse until a cookie dough consistency forms. Place into a bowl and set aside.

assemble: Arrange vegetables on a favorite large plate; get creative!

Put the dukkah and hummus in your favorite serving bowls and enjoy!

NOTE: My family just dips the veggies right in, but if you are serving guests you can put out small plates.

MIKE'S FAVORITE CHILI

My husband grew up on a meat-and-potatoes kind of diet. He's changed his ways since then but he still loves a good, hearty chili. This is something I made for him years ago when I was switching to a raw food diet and I wanted to help him lean vegan. He was in the military still and eating pretty poorly—think pizza, burgers, and burritos from wherever! He's never had to worry about weight, thanks to an extra-active metabolism, but I could see the whites of his eyes were in distress, and his overall emotional body was heavy. I kept adding in fresh kale salads and veggie-based dishes. I remember after two weeks of a plant-heavy diet, much had shifted for him emotionally and physically. That was the start to his lifestyle change, and this was a favorite from that time and still makes appearances in our house every other month or so! You can play with this recipe by adding in your favorite veggies and using up what's left in the refrigerator!

Makes 8 Servings

---

2 tablespoons coconut oil
1 red onion, diced
2 cups carrots, chopped
4 stalks of celery
½ jalapeño, minced
1 large yam, chopped
4 garlic cloves, minced
½ cup brown rice or quinoa
3 tablespoons chili powder
1 tablespoon cumin
2 cups tomatoes, diced (canned or fresh)
2 cups pure tomato sauce
2 (15 ounce) cans black beans
1 (15 ounce) can pinto or kidney beans
2 tablespoons rice wine vinegar
2 tablespoons maple syrup
1 cup water, optional
2 teaspoons pink salt
Fresh cilantro for topping

In a large soup pot, heat coconut oil over medium heat, then add in onion, carrots, celery, jalapeño, and yam. Sauté until onion is transparent and slightly crispy. Add the garlic and cook for 1 minute.

Add in the rice or quinoa, chili powder, and cumin, and stir well until combined.

Pour in diced tomatoes and tomato sauce, beans, vinegar, maple syrup, water if using, and salt. Bring to a boil, and then lower the heat and let simmer for about 1 hour.

Top with cilantro and enjoy!

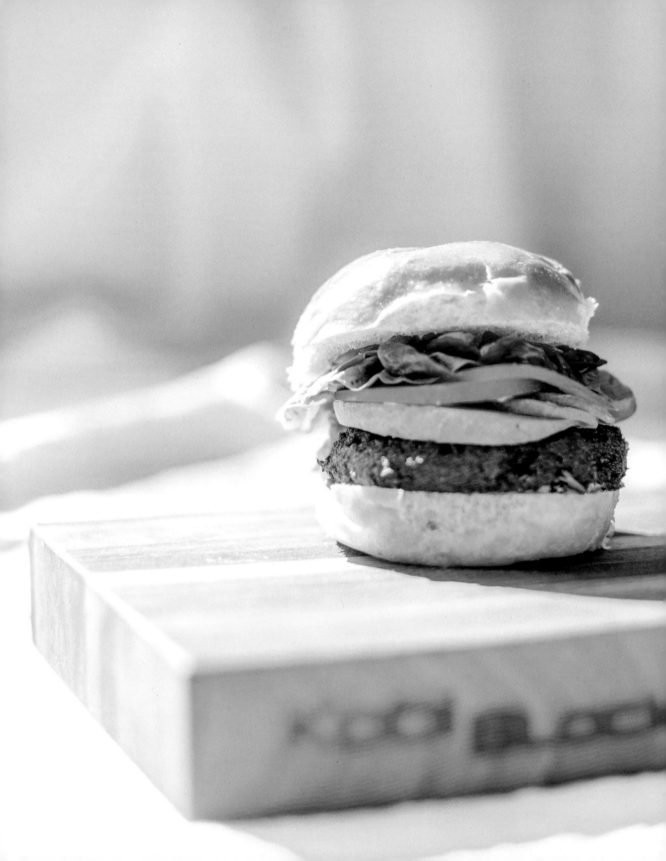

THE BEET BURGER

I typically don't like plant-based burgers. I was raised on Amy's veggie burgers, and just the thought makes my stomach hurt . . . but these are different. They are absolutely delightful in flavor and texture. They keep amazingly, too! I store them in the freezer and then cook them up for an easy yet impressive meal. Great on a bun, as the picture shows, but also good on a salad or even alone.

Makes 6 Patties

1 cup beets, peeled and diced (or shredded)
⅔ cup onion, chopped
1½ cup gluten-free oats
1 (16-oz can) chickpeas
¼ cup cassava or almond flour
1 small garlic clove
1 cup hemp seeds
½ cup flaxseed
⅛ cup coconut sugar
¼ teaspoon black pepper
2½ teaspoons cumin
2 tablespoons fresh or dried parsley
1 tablespoon coconut aminos
2 tablespoons coconut oil
5 teaspoons apple cider vinegar
1½ teaspoons salt

Preheat oven to 400°F.

Using an S blade in your food processor, combine all ingredients.

Process until a cookie-dough consistency forms.

Take mix out of the food processor and pour into a bowl. With your hands, form balls that are about 3 inches in diameter.

Line a baking sheet with parchment paper and then flatten the balls onto the sheet.

Bake for 25 minute or until solid, flipping once when half way through

NOTE: These burgers are great made the classic way as pictured or on a salad, I even eat them by themselves with some mustard when I'm in a hurry! They save well and will last up to a week in the refrigerator.

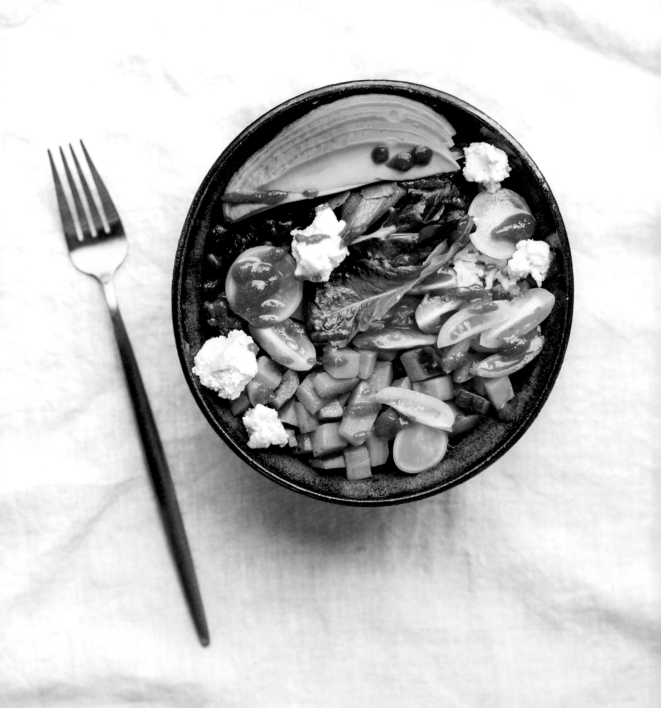

FIESTA BOWL

This is pretty much what I eat every night. I change it up here and there, but it's a go-to. Very simple and super filling. I make rice or quinoa two times a week so I always have it, I also always have beans soaking and ready to put in the slow cooker.

Makes 1 Serving

½ cup cooked quinoa or brown
   rice (page 273)
½ cup cooked black beans
   (page 267)
¼ avocado, sliced
1 cup romaine lettuce, chopped
¼ cup cilantro, minced
1 cup Yam Hash (page 157) or
   just a simple chopped yam
2 tablespoons cashew cheese
   (page 261)
¼ cup baby tomatoes, quartered

In a bowl, layer the quinoa and black beans on the bottom.

Then arrange the avocado, romaine lettuce, cilantro, Yam Hash, cheese, and tomatoes on top. Enjoy!

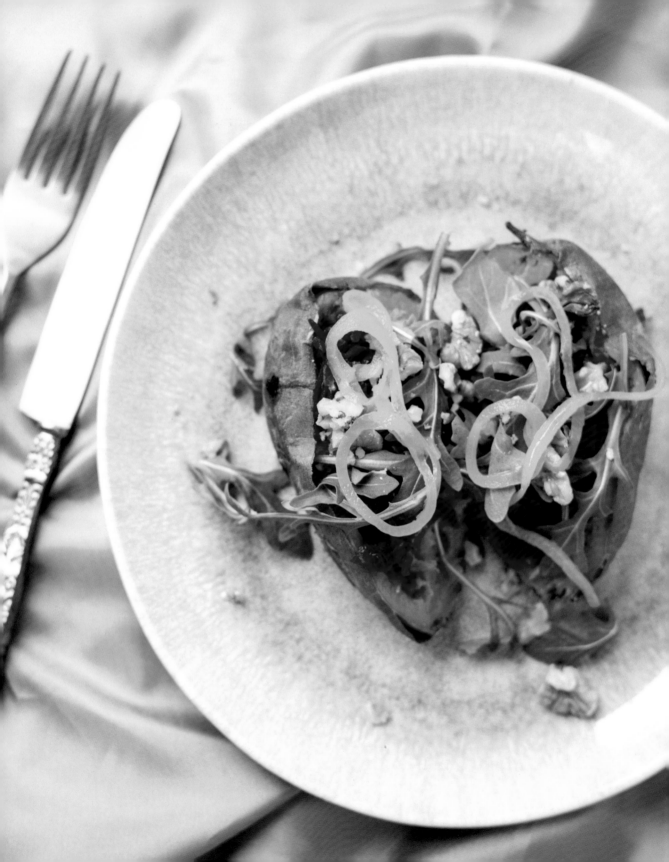

JUST A STUFFED YAM

This is another staple for dinnertime at my home. I love this during the change from summertime to autumn. You can really stuff it with whatever you love, but below is my go-to combo. The sauerkraut really balances out the flavor and gives it a nice boost as well as supporting your gut microbiome. Yams are wonderful for balancing your hormones and giving you good energy that is sustained over a long period of time.

Makes 1 Serving

---

1 medium yam
1 tablespoon coconut oil
Pinch of salt
¼ cup favorite sauerkraut
1 tablespoon Onion Turmeric
  Pickles (page 255)
1 cup arugula, chopped
6 walnuts, crushed
2 tablespoons favorite dressing
  (see pages 222–225 for ideas)

Bake your yam of choice. I usually bake mine at 400°F. for about 45 minutes, depending on the size.

Take it out and cut it in two. Mash up the inside with coconut oil and a pinch of salt, leaving the outside intact.

Top with sauerkraut, pickled onions, arugula, walnuts, and your favorite dressing.

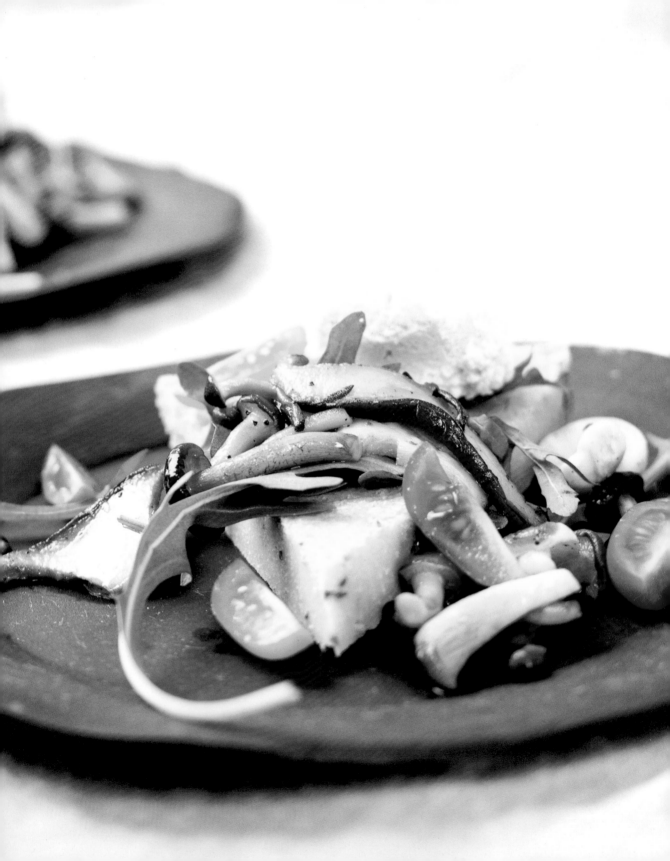

SOCCA PANCAKE WITH SAUTEED MUSHROOMS + MACADAMIA NUT BUTTER

The base of this recipe is exactly like the Socca Pancake on page 141. I originally got inspired to play with chickpeas from the beautiful and talented ladies from Cap Beauty, Cindy DiPrima Morisse and Kerrilynn Pamer. Their book *Transformational Beauty* has some amazing recipes worth playing with—the book is also a work of art. It's a must-see. Anyway, they inspired the chickpea socca pancake recipes I've been playing with. I'm grateful, because I don't eat many eggs personally, although my son and husband love them. I like to add this dish in once in a while for them to change it up and give their bodies a break from the eggs. They both love it, and I get to enjoy it with them.

Makes 4 Servings

Socca, from page 141

topping

2 tablespoons butter, ghee, or coconut oil
1 shallot, minced
6 cups sliced, assorted mushrooms (such as shiitake, oyster, morel, chanterelle, cremini)
Salt and black pepper to taste
2 cups arugula, loosely packed
1 cup baby tomatoes, quartered
½ cup macadamia nut butter page 261)
Black truffle oil (optional but amazing)

make the topping: In a skillet, melt the butter, ghee, or coconut oil, then add in the shallot and cook for 3 minutes.

Add the mushrooms and cook for about 5 minutes, stirring occasionally.

Once they release their juices and start to brown, add in the salt and pepper. Let cook a little longer, then set aside.

assemble: Cut socca like a pie, and place slices on plates. Add on a scoop of mushrooms, arugula, baby tomatoes, macadamia nut butter, and then top with truffle oil.

Serve and enjoy!

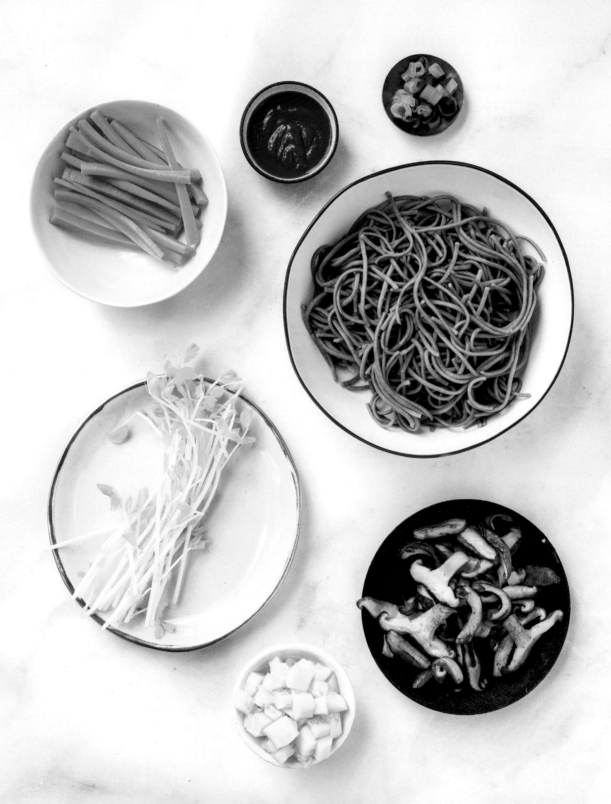

BUCKWHEAT RAMEN BOWL

It took me a while to hop on the ramen train, but once I got on, I realized I'd been missing out! Making healthy versions of this comforting meal has become a fun interactive family meal! My son loves to add in ideas. Play and have fun, there are no rules with this.

Makes 2 Servings

---

1 pack buckwheat noodles (I love Eden selected 100% buckwheat soba noodles)
1 cup shiitake mushrooms, sliced
2 medium bok choy, bottom sliced off
2 tablespoons coconut oil
4 tablespoons ponzu sauce, divided
3 cups bone or vegetable broth
4 chives, diced
2 carrots, julienned
1 small handful of pea or bean sprouts
½ cup crushed pistachios or almonds
2 eggs, boiled (optional)
Sriracha
Salt and pepper, to taste

NOTE: You can make this your own and add all types of veggies! So much fun.

Cook noodles per package instructions, rinse, and cool. Set aside.

Sauté shiitakes and bok choy in 2 tablespoons coconut oil and 2 tablespoons ponzu sauce. They should be nice and crisp, which takes about 10 minutes.

Boil broth until nice and hot.

Get two of your favorite bowls, and place the noodle in the bottoms, then pour the broth around the noodles.

Place the sautéed bok choy and shiitake in the broth and top with chives, carrots, sprouts, nuts, and sriracha, and then top with remaining ponzu sauce.

Slice the boiled egg, if using, and place into the bowl.

Salt and pepper to taste.

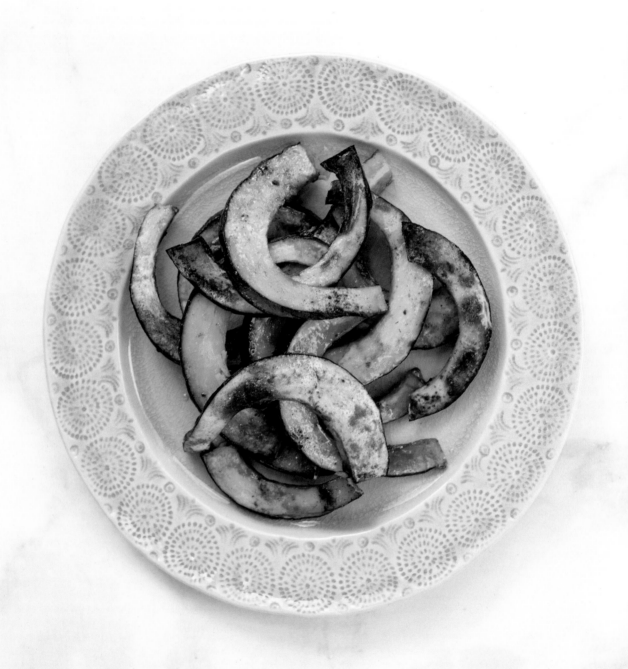

CINNAMON + MAPLE ROASTED KABOCHA SQUASH

For some this may be an excellent side dish, but for me it's a whole meal. I love it. Kabocha squash is so filling and rich, it's great for cold nights. You can eat it sweet or savory and it goes well with just about anything. You can really use any kind of squash for this recipe!

Makes 2 Servings

---

1 kabocha squash
¼ cup pastured butter, ghee, or
   coconut oil
3 tablespoons maple syrup
1 teaspoon cinnamon
½ teaspoon pink salt

Preheat oven to 400°F.

Cut squash into four large pieces, remove seeds, and then slice in to ¼-inch slices. Place on a large baking sheet.

In a small saucepan, melt your butter or oil. Pour over the squash along with the maple syrup. Sprinkle with cinnamon and salt, then place in the oven for 30 minutes until nice and toasty brown.

THE WEEKDAY MEAL

This is my quickest most easy to make weekday meal. It does require that you have cooked quinoa or rice on hand as well as a baked yam. I like to batch cook these things early in the week so they are available for easy meals like this one. You could also use buckwheat or any favorite grain or seed.

Makes 2 Servings

¼ onion, diced
2 tablespoons coconut oil
1 cup cooked grain (such as rice
   or quinoa) or seed
2 cups shredded kale
2 cup spinach
1 cup baked yam, chopped
2 eggs (optional)
Salt
Pepper

Sauté onion in coconut oil in a medium-sized skillet until golden.

Add in grain, kale, spinach, and yam, and cook until kale is soft. Use a spatula to keep from sticking to the pan.

Add in eggs if you choose and scramble into the mix. Salt and pepper to taste!

LETTUCE WRAP TACOS

These are so fun and super healthy. Perfect for people who don't want to give up taco Tuesday, but also want to stay high vibe. The walnut chorizo it what we make at Local Juicery, and every Tuesday we sell out. These plant-powered tacos are filling and absolutely delicious.

Makes 8 Servings

---

wraps

8 romaine lettuce leaves

filling

1 cup baby tomatoes, quartered
1 avocado, thinly sliced
½ cup cilantro, stems removed
½ cup Cashew Cheese (page 261)
4 cups Easy Black Beans
  (page 267)

walnut chorizo

2 cups walnuts
2 teaspoons chipotle powder
2 teaspoons cumin powder
½ teaspoon salt
¼ cup nutritional yeast
¼ cup extra-virgin olive oil

Wash, dry, and lay out 8 large romaine lettuce leaves. Prep all the ingredients for the filling and set aside.

make the walnut chorizo: Using the S blade on your food processor, combine walnuts, chipotle powder, cumin, salt, nutritional yeast, and olive oil.

Pulse until sticky but not mushy—it should have a nutty consistency.

assemble: Place a dried romaine leaf on a cutting board, layer with tomatoes, avocado, cilantro, cashew cheese, black beans, and chorizo. Fold and enjoy!

NOTE: You can prep some of the ingredients the day before! I always make a big batch of cashew cheese and black beans at the beginning of the week so I can easily put these together.

A FEW DELICIOUS DRESSINGS

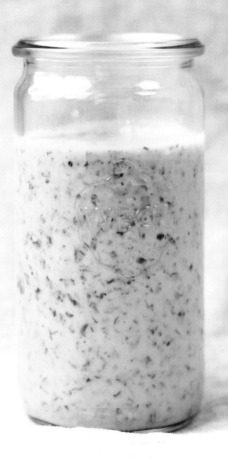

CLASSIC GREEN GODDESS

This is a great dressing for salads, but also a wonderful sauce for dipping veggies, chips, or topping your baked yam. It's so creamy and flavorful. Check out Coconut Cult yogurt or Living Cultures coconut yogurt, which are raw and bursting with active and alive probiotics.
Makes 4 Servings

6 ounces coconut yogurt
1 cup cilantro, stems removed
2 tablespoons minced leek
1 large lemon or lime, freshly squeezed
2 tablespoons raw honey
¼ cup extra-virgin olive oil
½ teaspoon garlic powder
¼ cup water
½ teaspoon salt

Combine all ingredients in a blender and blend until well combined. Add more water if you find it's too thick.

Keeps well for about a week when sealed tightly in a jar in the refrigerator.

HONEY MUSTARD VINAGERETTE

This can make any bland salad burst with flavor. It's simple to make and really delicious. I've yet to find a salad that it doesn't taste great on.
Makes 1 Serving

3 tablespoons Dijon mustard
5 tablespoons apple cider vinegar
3 tablespoons raw honey
¾ cup extra-virgin olive oil
½ teaspoon salt
¼ cup water

Combine all ingredients in a blender and blend on high until perfectly creamy.

Keeps well for about a week when sealed tightly in a jar in the refrigerator.

SUMMER'S CAESAR

During my last pregnancy, I had such a hard time getting greens in during the first trimester. I could barely stand the thought of broccoli! This was the only thing I could eat that was green. I would literally dream about it. I did add parmesan to my version when pregnant but you can keep this salad vegan by making your own vegan parmesan! All you have do to is grate macadamia nuts, it makes an amazing vegan parmesan.

Makes 4 Servings

¼ cup extra-virgin olive oil
4 tablespoons water
2 lemons, juiced
1 tablespoon Worcestershire
  sauce
1 tablespoon Dijon mustard
½ garlic clove
1 date, pitted
⅓ cup pepitas
1 tablespoon capers
1 teaspoon onion powder
1 teaspoon kelp flakes
Pinch of pink salt

Combine all ingredients in a blender and blend on high until perfectly creamy.

Pour into a mason jar. Keeps for about 1 week in the refrigerator

CARROT-GINGER DRESSING

This recipe is inspired by Gwyneth Paltrow from her book, *It's All Good*—I got obsessed and started making it every day. Eventually I changed it up a bit to fit my needs.
Makes About 1 Cup

4 carrots, peeled and chopped
1 small shallot, peeled
⅓ cup fresh ginger, chopped
2 tablespoons miso
¼ cup rice vinegar
2 tablespoons raw honey
3 tablespoons sesame oil
⅓ cup water
½ teaspoon pink salt

Combine all ingredients in a blender and pulse until well combined. There should be a bit of texture, not smooth and creamy.

Pour into a mason jar. Keeps for about 1 week in the refrigerator

PLANT RANCH

The essential dressing. I like it on every type of salad.
Makes About 1 Cup

½ cup Cashew Crema (page 259)
2 tablespoons minced chives
½ garlic clove, minced
1 teaspoon onion powder
1 tablespoon lemon juice
1 tablespoon parsley, minced
2 tablespoons dill, minced
¼ cup water or almond milk
¼ teaspoon pink salt

Combine all ingredients in a blender and blend on high until perfectly creamy.

Pour into a mason jar. Keeps for about 1 week in the refrigerator

LEMON TAHINI

Everyone has a version of Lemon Tahini dressing! I like mine with a little spice and sweet. The cumin and honey add a unique spin to this classic.

Makes 2 Servings

4 tablespoon tahini
1 small garlic clove, minced
4 tablespoons lemon, freshly
    squeezed
⅓ cup extra-virgin olive oil
2 teaspoons raw honey (optional)
¼ teaspoon cumin
½ teaspoon pink salt
¼ cup water

Whisk all ingredients together in a small bowl until very smooth.

Keeps well for about a week when sealed tightly in a jar in the refrigerator.

NOTE: You can also put it into the blender if you can't get the tahini to smooth out. Another trick is using hot water instead of cold.

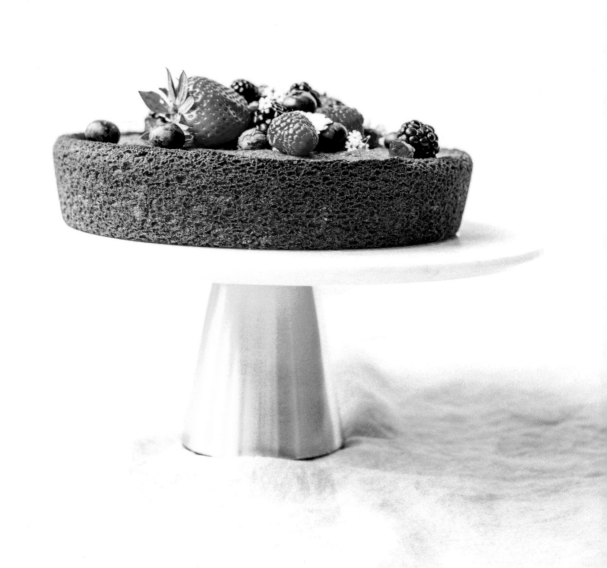

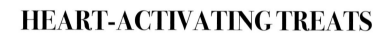

HEART-ACTIVATING TREATS

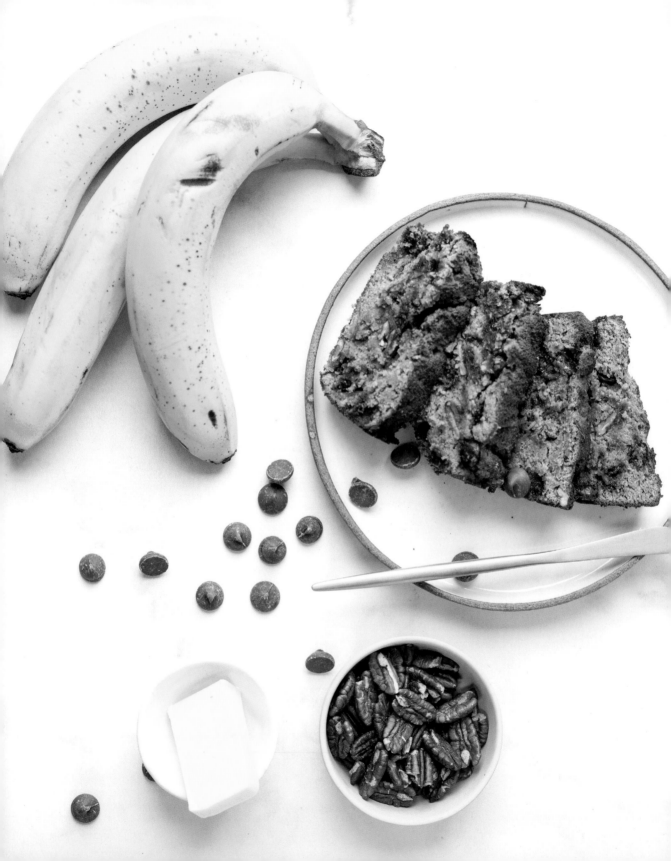

CHOCOLATE PROTEIN BANANA BREAD

Like grandma made, but loaded with superfoods and grain-free! This banana bread is just the right amount of good gooey and then you get the nice crunch from the pecans. The chocolate chips melt in your mouth. You'll be in banana bread heaven. I love slicing it and putting a nice pat of grass-fed butter on it, or you can smother in almond butter or coconut oil. Just as delicious. Indulge without one ounce of guilt, because life is too short. Best to share with your most loved ones.

Makes 1 Loaf

Coconut oil, for the pan
1½ cup smashed bananas, about
   3 medium bananas
¼ cup almond butter
1 tablespoon almond extract
1 teaspoon vanilla extract
2 eggs
¾ teaspoon salt
⅛ cup coconut sugar
¾ cup coconut flour
1 cup almond flour
¾ teaspoon baking soda
¾ cup chocolate chips
⅓ cup crushed pecans

Preheat oven to 375°F. and coat an 8 x 4-inch loaf pan with coconut oil and a light dusting of almond flour.

In a blender, combine bananas, almond butter, almond extract, vanilla, eggs, salt, and coconut sugar. Blend until smooth.

In a medium bowl combine almond flour, coconut flour, and baking soda. Whisk until well mixed.

Pour wet mix into the dry flour mix and stir. Then fold in chocolate chips and pecans.

Pour mixture into bread pan. Bake for 40 minutes. Then remove bread, cool a bit, then remove from the pan and let cool all the way.

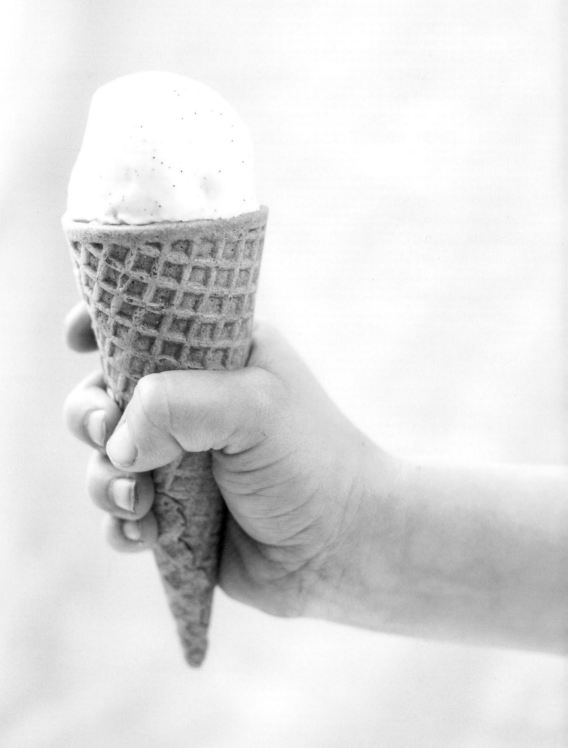

VANILLA ICE CREAM

Ice cream is such a love of mine, but milk, sugar, and I don't get along at all. So thankfully there is this decadent goodness that actually tastes better to me than any other ice cream, because I know it's actually good for me. Zero guilt. I love adding chai spice or chocolate to this for different flavors. So many fun ways to make it your own! However, you will need an ice cream maker to bring this deliciousness to life.

Makes 4 Servings

2 cups young coconut meat
1 cup cashews, soaked
¾ cup maple syrup
4 tablespoons vanilla extract
½ cup coconut water
½–1 teaspoon salt

Blend all ingredients in a high-speed blender until delightfully creamy.

Pour into ice cream maker, following instructions.

NOTE: You can play with flavoring this! Just remember that you'll need more than you think with flavors.

CARDAMOM LIME GELATO

This isn't really gelato in the traditional sense, but it's so creamy and amazing that it might as well be. You will need an ice cream maker for this recipe, and it's worth it! I love this recipe alongside the Chocolate Protein Banana Bread on page 229. Enjoy this all vegan and raw treat.

Makes 1 Serving

3 cups young coconut meat
1 cups cashews, soaked
1½ cups coconut oil
3 tablespoons vanilla extract
2 cups maple syrup
1 teaspoon salt
2 teaspoons cardamom
¾ cup lime juice
2 tablespoons lime zest

Combine all ingredients in a blender and blend on high until perfectly creamy.

Follow your ice cream maker instructions to pour the liquid in.

It should be thick and creamy when finished.

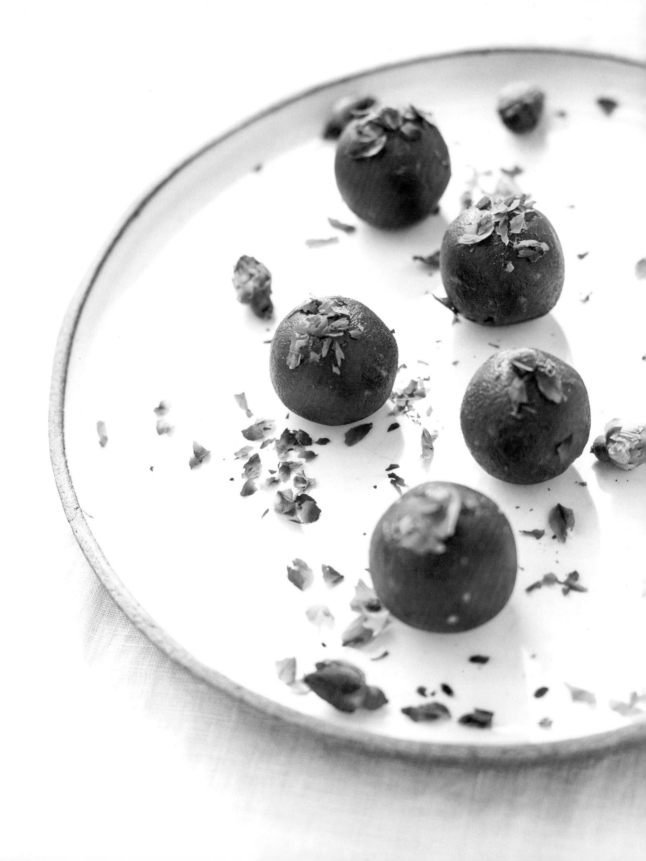

CASHEW TRUFFLES

These are a total hit in my house. I've actually had to hide them so they don't all get eaten up at once. My mom especially loves these, and I consider her a chocolate connoisseur. It's likely your whole family will be munching these down quicker than you can roll them.

Makes About 18 Truffles

---

truffles

1 cup raw cashew butter
½ cup maple syrup
2 teaspoons vanilla
½ cup cacao butter, melted
¾ teaspoon salt
1 cup raw cacao powder

topping suggestions

Rose petals
Cacao powder
Cinnamon and coconut sugar
Crushed pistachios
Raw shredded coconut

In a high-speed blender or food processor, combine cashew butter, maple syrup, vanilla, melted cacao butter, and salt. Make sure not to overprocess, as the oil from the cacao butter will separate.

Once well combined, add in the cacao powder.

Put the mix into a large bowl and refrigerate until solid.

Use an ice cream scoop to scoop out tablespoon-sized truffles and then roll them with your hands to get them perfectly round.

Top as desired and enjoy!

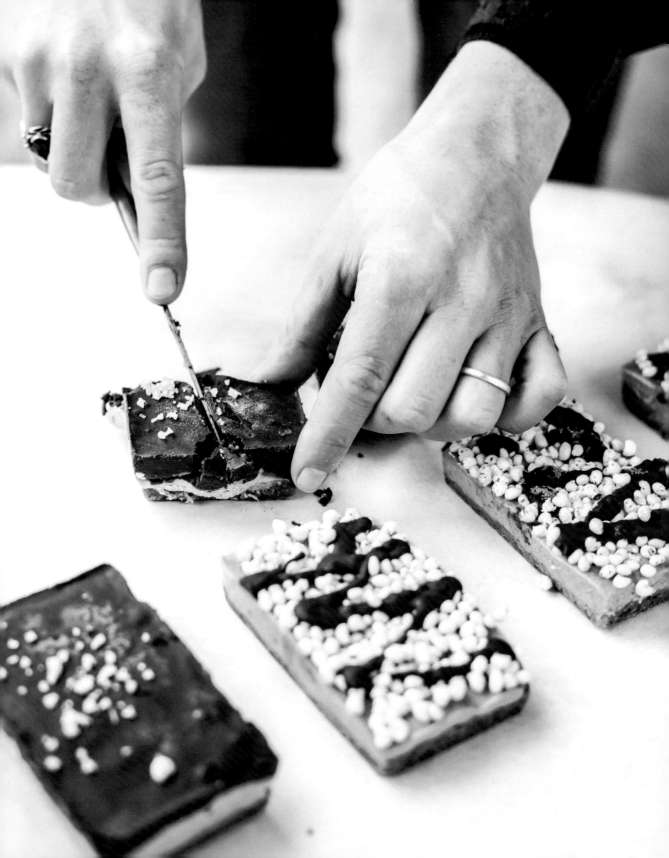

CARAMEL CANDY BARS

Sometimes you just need a little oxytocin in the form of chocolate. This homemade chocolate and silky date caramel will do the trick. Great for birthday parties, potluck, or just having on hand for those moments of need.

Makes 9 Bars

---

crust
2 cups pecans
4 dates, pitted
⅓ cup coconut oil
1 tablespoon vanilla extract
¼ teaspoon pink salt

filling
9 dates, pitted
½ cup coconut oil
¾ cup cashews, soaked
1 vanilla bean, scraped
¼ cup water
1 cup puffed millet cereal

topping
1⅔ cup cacao butter
1½ cup cacao powder
1½ cup maple syrup
½ teaspoon pink salt

make the crust: Lightly oil a silicone baking mold (preferably 2.5" x 1.5" x .75") with coconut oil.

Combine all crust ingredients in a food processor until smooth. Divide the crust into each mold and press with fingers until flat. Put into the refrigerator while you make the filling.

make the filling: In a blender, combine dates, coconut oil, cashew, vanilla bean, and water. Blend until incredibly creamy!

Pour the creamy mixture into each mold, about ¼ cup per mold, then top each one with puffed millet.

make the topping: In a saucepan, slowly melt cacao butter on low. Once melted, sift in cacao powder using a fine-mesh strainer. Then add maple syrup and salt and whisk together.

Pour chocolate topping on bars, Return to the freezer to chill for 30 minutes.

Once they are chilled, they pop right out of the molds for you to enjoy!

NOTE: I used 2.5" x 1.5" x .75" silicone molds for this recipe. You can find them online, or better yet, look at your local cooking store.

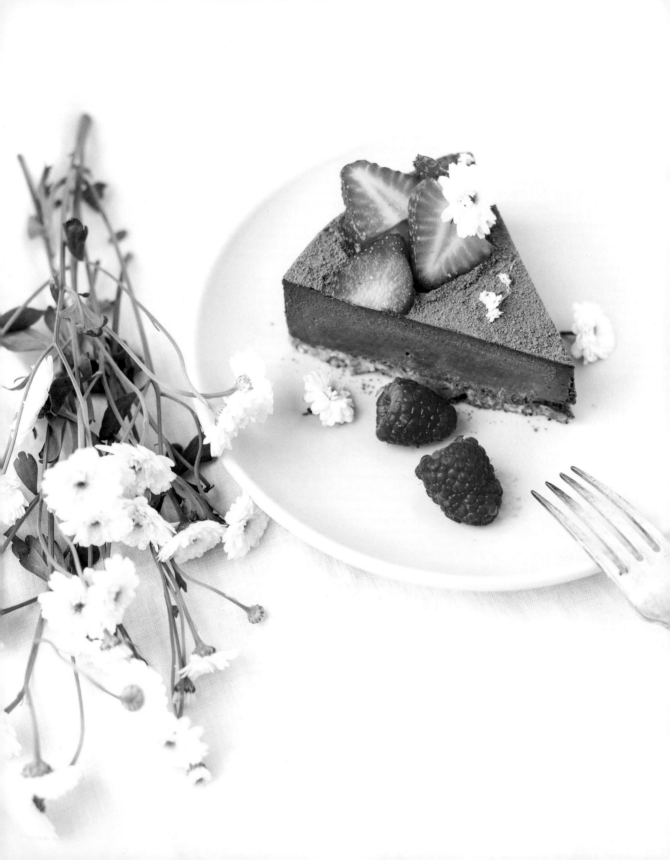

CHOCOLATE HAZELNUT TART

This is by far my favorite chocolate dessert. I adore hazelnuts and everything about them. This isn't 100 percent raw because of the roasted hazelnuts, but other than that it's all glowy goodness. I love making this for holidays and surprising guests with how healthy it is. No one ever knows—they typically think it's a play on traditional flourless chocolate cake.

Makes a 9-Inch Pie

crust
1½ cups roasted hazelnuts
⅛ cup coconut oil
⅛ cup maple syrup
¼ teaspoon pink salt

filling
1½ cups soaked hazelnuts
2 cups soaked cashews
1⅓ cup maple syrup
1¼ cup cacao powder
¾ cup coconut oil
1 teaspoon pink salt

NOTE: If you are roasting your own hazelnuts, line a baking sheet with parchment paper and add your hazelnuts. Bake at 350°F for 5 to 10 minutes, keeping a close eye on them.

make the crust: Line a 9-inch springform pan with plastic wrap and set aside.

Combine all crust ingredients in a food processor and blend until a cookie dough consistency forms. Press the crust into the bottom of the pan until flat and even. Set in the freezer while you make the filling.

make the filling: In a high-speed blender, combine all filling ingredients and blend until incredibly creamy. You'll have to stop the blender every so often and scrape the sides with a spatula. The air bubbles that form will also have to be moved with a spatula.

Once your filling is dreamy and creamy, take out the crust and pour the filling in. Bang on the counter a few times to even it out.

Place in the freezer for at least an hour to assist it in setting up. It can stay here for as long as you need! Up to 3 months if sealed with plastic wrap.

When you are ready to enjoy, let thaw and then sift cacao powder on top. Serve with favorite berries or more toasted hazelnuts.

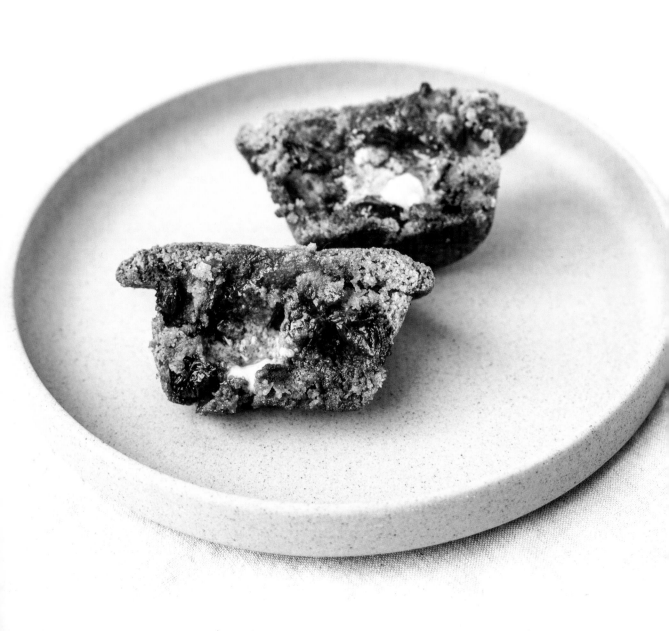

CLASSIC BLUEBERRY MUFFINS

There is simply nothing better. I've tried many a recipe in search of a muffin that was gluten-free and fabulous. I drew inspiration from multiple recipes to create this one. I think it has to do with the almond extract, it somehow brings out the blueberry flavor and creates a unique spin on a classic. I think you're going to love it.

Makes 9 Muffins

⅓ cup pastured butter, room temperature
¾ cup maple syrup
½ cup full fat coconut milk
2 eggs
1 tablespoon vanilla extract
1 tablespoon almond extract
1½ cups almond flour
1¼ cups brown rice flour
¼ cup arrowroot
1 teaspoon salt
½ teaspoon baking powder
½ teaspoon baking soda
1¼ cups blueberries, fresh or frozen

Preheat the oven to 350°F.

In a bowl, combine butter, maple syrup, and coconut milk, and cream together with a mixer. Add in eggs, vanilla and almond extract

In a separate bowl, combine almond flour, rice flour, arrowroot, salt, baking powder, and baking soda. Mix well.

Add the wet mix to the dry mix and stir until combined. Fold in blueberries.

Line a muffin tin with 12 muffin liners, and fill with the batter. Sprinkle the remaining coconut sugar on top of each muffin. Bake for 25 minutes or until a toothpick comes out clean.

Cool before eating if you can wait!

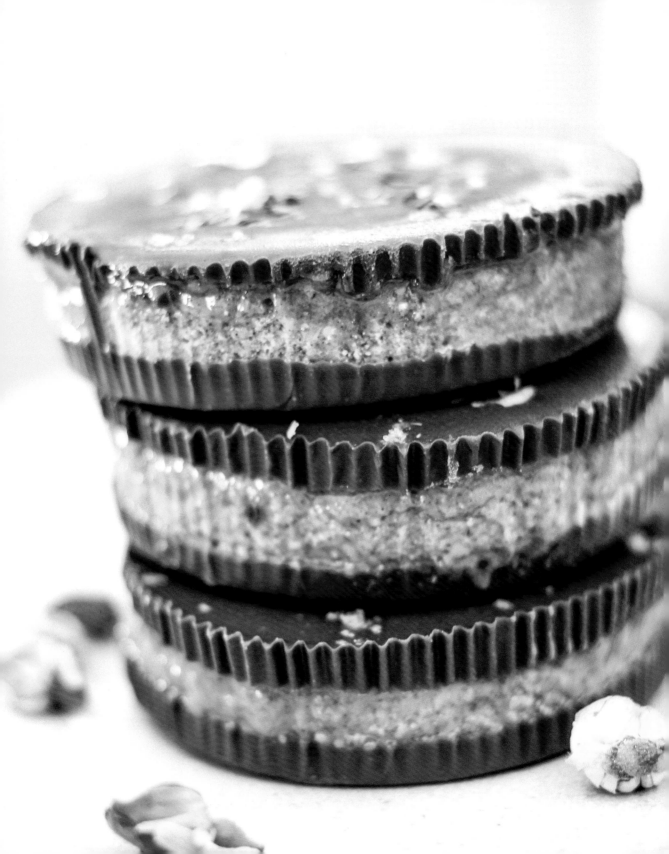

CHOCOLATE CORDYCEPS + ROSE BARS

Chocolate, roses, and cordyceps caramel are meant to go together. Just wait and see! This recipe takes a little time, but it's very much worth the effort. These bars are dreamy! They keep well in the freezer for later enjoyment. I add rose absolute oil to this recipe, but you can omit it if you don't have it on hand.

Makes 12 Bars

chocolate layers

9 ounces chocolate chips
2 tablespoons maple syrup
⅓ cup stone-ground almond butter
3 tablespoons coconut oil
1 teaspoon vanilla extract
5 drops rose absolute oil
¼ teaspoon salt

filling

¾ cup stone-ground almond butter
1 teaspoon vanilla extract
1 tablespoon maple syrup
2 tablespoons brown rice syrup
1 teaspoon cordyceps mushroom powder
2 tablespoons water
¼ teaspoon salt

make the chocolate: Line a mini muffin tin with muffin liners. Set aside.

In a double boiler, combine all chocolate layer ingredients. Heat until all is melted together.

Pour about 3 tablespoons of melted chocolate into each muffin liner. Reserve enough chocolate for the topping as well.

Place in the freezer after you fill.

Keep the remainder of the chocolate on in the double builder so it stays a liquid.

make the filling: In a saucepan, add all filling ingredients. Stir continuously, letting the mixture warm up and liquify.

Remove from heat and quickly bring out the chocolate layer from the freezer.

assemble: Pour about 3 tablespoons of the warmed almond butter filling into the chocolate muffin liners. Then return to the freezer for 10 minutes.

Remove muffin tin from the freezer and divide the remainder of the chocolate onto each. Top with rose petals and return to the freezer for another 10 minutes. Then they're ready to eat!

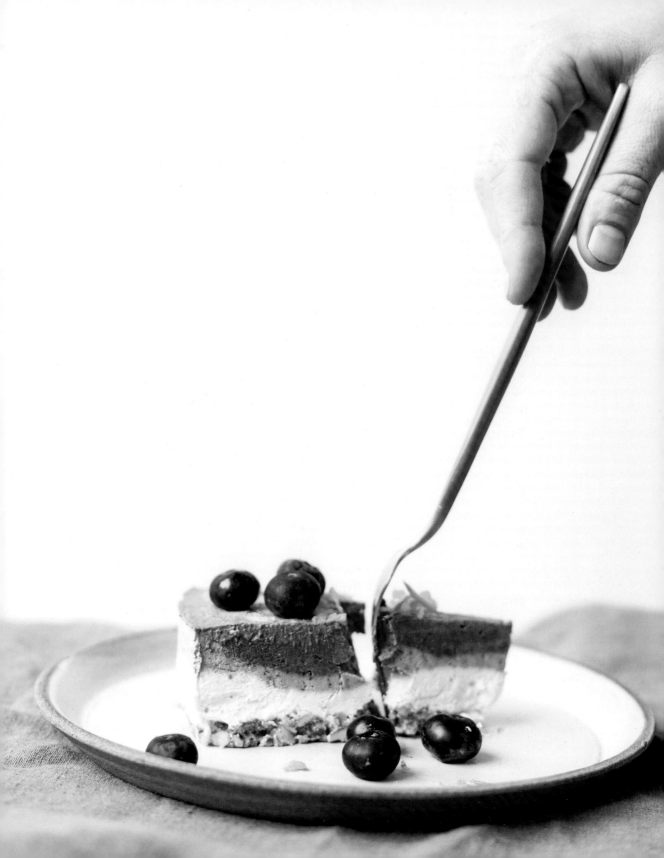

RAW BLUEBERRY LEMON LAYER CAKE

Blueberries and cream have a special place in my heart. When I was a little girl I had a book called *When the Sun Rose*. In one part there is a beautiful picture of a little girl and an imaginary lion eating blueberries and cream, and I have loved it ever since. If you have kiddos, you should definitely get the book! This recipe is blueberries and cream perfected. The lemon gives it a slight tart taste that is reminiscent of classic cheesecakes. The layers and bleeding of color makes this a wonderful treat for serving to guests. Plating of this cake can be fun, too; let frozen berries melt all over and create a messy but beautiful piece of cake art! Enjoy.

Makes a 9-Inch Pie

crust
1½ cups walnuts or almonds
¼ cup coconut oil
3 tablespoons maple syrup
1 teaspoon vanilla extract
1 teaspoon almond extract
2 tablespoons lemon zest
¼ teaspoon pink slat

filling
3 cups soaked cashew
¾ cup raw honey
¾ cup lemon juice
3 tablespoons lemon zest
1 cup coconut oil
⅓ cup water
¾ teaspoon pink salt
2 tablespoons vanilla
1 tablespoon almond extract
2½ cups frozen blueberries
(frozen is best for this recipe)

NOTE: I love Vitamix for raw cakes such as this. They are really strong and give a nice, smooth texture.

make the crust: Line a 9-inch springform pan with plastic wrap and set aside.

Combine all crust ingredients in a food processor and blend until a cookie dough consistency forms.

Press the crust into the bottom of the pan until flat and even. Set in the freezer while you move on to the filling.

make the filling: In a high-speed blender, combine all ingredients except blueberries. Blend until incredibly creamy—up to 3 minutes may be necessary depending on your blender. You'll have to stop the blender every so often and scrape the sides with a spatula. The air bubbles that form will also have to be moved with a spatula.

Pour ⅓ of the filling into the pie crust and move to the refrigerator.

Add 1 cup of the frozen blueberries into the remaining filling and blend. Pour ½ of the now purple filling over the first layer of white filling and smooth. Return to freezer.

Pour the remaining blueberries into the filling and blend. Bring out the cake and top with this dark purple layer. Cover with plastic wrap and let chill for at least 2 hours before serving.

Top with assorted berries and enjoy!

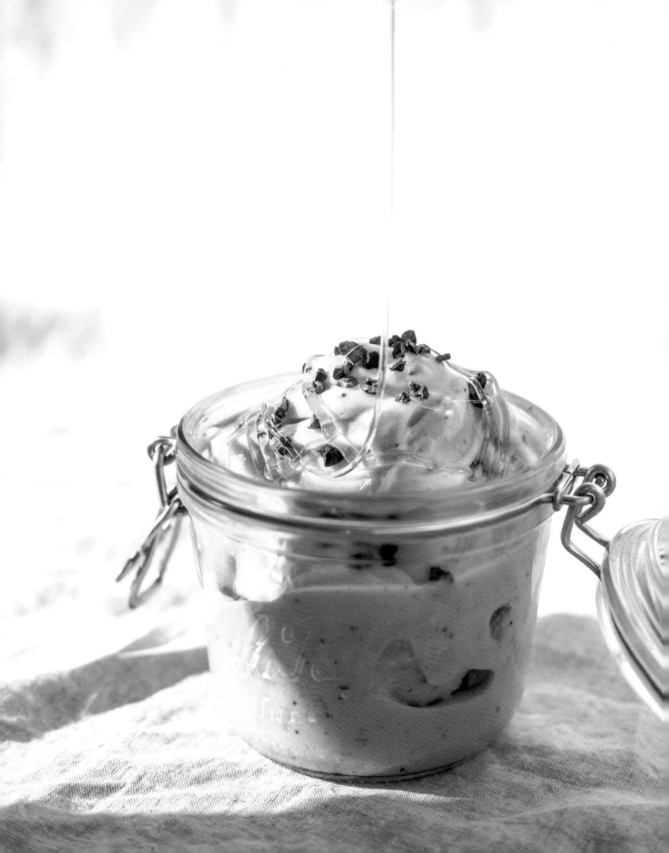

BANANA NICE CREAM

My first memory of this amazing stuff was in the 1980s at our farm in Missouri. My mom had a Champion juicer and one day decided to put frozen bananas though it. Mind blown. She topped it with raisins and, as a three-year-old, it was literally the best thing I had ever had. I've updated the recipe a bit and you don't have to have a Champion juicer for the amazing alternative ice cream, just a good blender. You can add all sorts of fun things to this recipe. I love adding cacao powder or almond butter and making it a little extra thick and creamy, but give the simple version a try too, it's marvelous on its own as well. The perfect summertime treat.
Makes 2 Servings

3–4 ripe bananas, peeled and
  sliced
Large pinch pink salt
½ teaspoon vanilla extract
2 teaspoons maple syrup or
  honey (optional)

toppings and blended ideas
2 tablespoons cacao powder
  added into mix
½ cup crushed pecans stirred in
Cacao nibs (as pictured)
Fresh fruit
Stone-ground almond butter

Freeze the sliced bananas in ziplock bags or on a baking tray. It's best to do this one day ahead of making.

Once the bananas are frozen solid, combine bananas, salt, vanilla, and maple syrup in a blender.

Blend until very creamy, put into your favorite bowl, and top with all your favorite things.

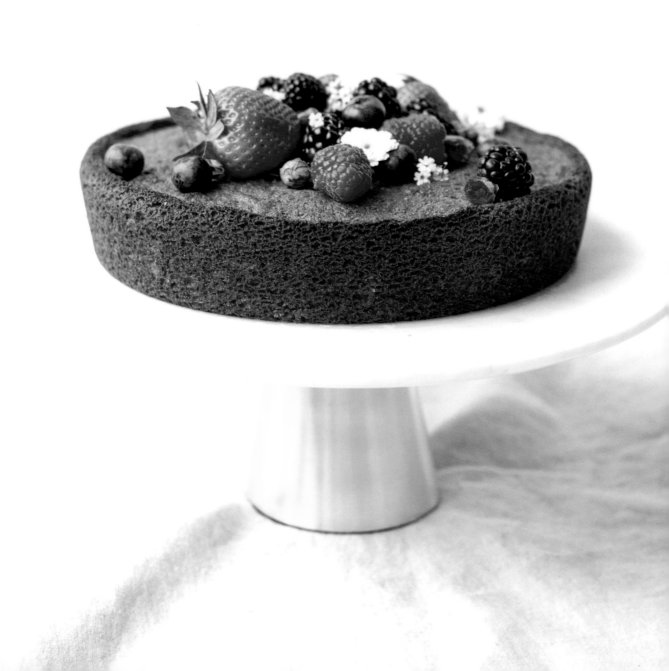

BIRTHDAY POUND CAKE

You won't believe how amazingly delicious this cake is. It's so moist, so perfectly sweet, and satisfying to all! It's similar to traditional pound cake but without the processed sugar, gluten, or cream. I do use butter in this recipe, but see the Note just in case you need to omit it.

Makes 1 9-Inch Cake

cake

2 cups almond flour
½ cup coconut flour
1 teaspoon baking soda
¼ cup arrowroot
½ teaspoon salt
¼ coconut sugar
¾ maple syrup
6 tablespoons butter, room temperature
⅔ cup coconut oil
2 teaspoons almond extract
½ cup almond milk
4 eggs

Preheat oven to 350°F.

Combine almond flour, coconut flour, baking soda, arrow root, and salt in a large mixing bowl. Mix well and set aside.

In a separate mixing bowl, combine coconut sugar, maple syrup, butter, coconut oil, almond extract, almond milk, and eggs.

Oil your 9-inch cake pan with coconut oil and a light dusting of coconut flour. Pour in the batter.

Bake for 35 minutes or until a toothpick inserted in the center comes out clean.

Let cool all the way, then remove from the pan.

NOTE: You can omit butter in this recipe, just add an additional ¼ cup coconut oil. If you want to make layers, double or even triple the recipe!

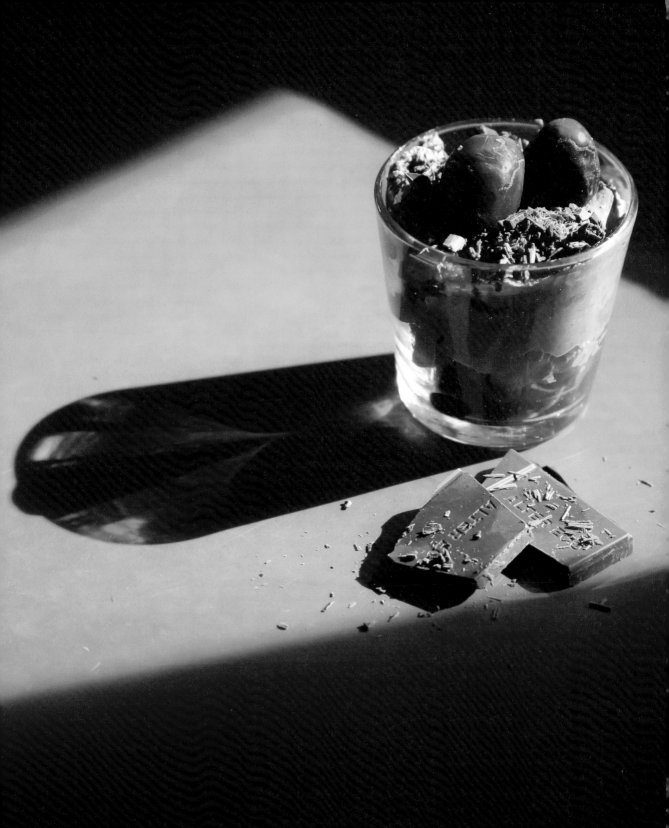

CHOCOLATE MOUSSE

One of the main ingredients in this dreamy mousse is avocado, but you'd never know it. It's incredibly silky and rich and makes you feel like you're doing something super naughty. But you're not. Just enjoy.

Makes 8–10 Servings

8 avocados, pitted
1½ cups coconut oil
2 cups cashews, soaked
1½ cups water
2½–3 cups raw cacao powder
1 vanilla bean, scraped
1½ cups maple syrup
1 teaspoon salt

Combine avocado meat, coconut oil, cashews, and water in a high-speed blender. You'll need to stop it occasionally to scrape the sides with a spatula and pop the air bubbles that can keep the blender from catching.

Once your mixture is incredibly smooth, transfer to a large food processor, working in two batches if necessary.

Once have your avocado mixture in the food processor, add in the cacao powder, vanilla bean, maple syrup, and salt. Process until well combined and very creamy.

Pour into your favorite tumbler and top with fresh fruit and any other favorite toppings.

Keeps well for up to 1 week in the refrigerator. You can also freeze it! Great for at least 2 months when frozen.

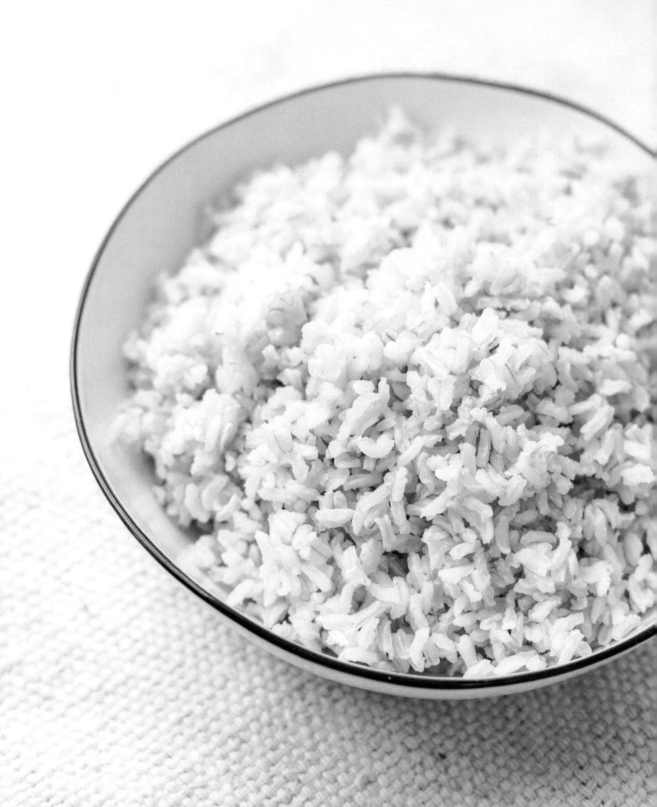

BASIC GROUNDING RECIPES

PERFECT BROWN RICE OR QUINOA

The perfect rice or quinoa has surprisingly been the biggest hurdle for me to get over. It's the simple things that sometimes are the hardest! I think it's because I'm impatient, I'm always opening the lid too early and I could never just commit to measuring the water, I always wanted to free pour. I finally broke some bad habits and discovered the perfect ratios.
Makes 6 Servings

2 cups quinoa or rice
2½ cups water
1 tablespoon coconut oil
   (optional)
1 teaspoon salt

Bring the water to a boil and then add in the quinoa or rice, coconut oil, and salt

Cover with a lid and bring to a boil again, and then lower the temperature to low. Cook until the water is gone, roughly 35 minutes.

NOTE: A note on elevation and climate: if you are at higher elevation or in drier climates, you may need ¼–½ cup more water. If you are sea level and in a moist client, you may subtract ¼–½ cup water.

BASIC LENTILS

I love lentils as an add-on to almost anything. You can use them in salad, as a side, in soup, add them to breads or baked goods, add to scrambles—the options are endless! It's important to soak them or buy them sprouted at your local health food store. See the soaking chart on page 279.
Makes 2 Servings

4 cups water
1½ cups lentils, soaked
1 teaspoon salt
1 tablespoon coconut oil
   (optional)

Bring the water to a boil and then add in the lentils.

Cover with a lid and bring to a boil again and then lower the temperature to low.

Cook until the water is gone, about 45 minutes.

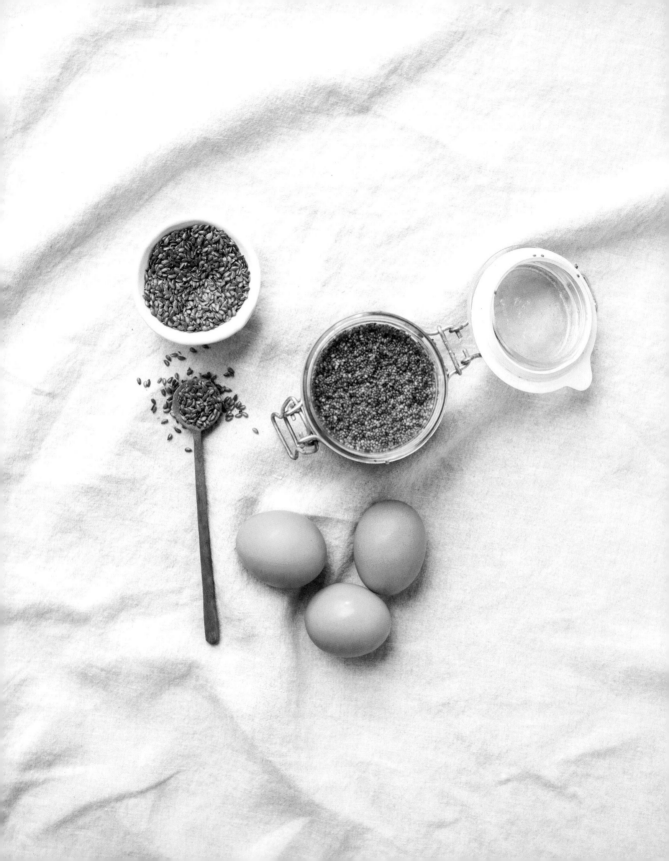

CHIA OR FLAX EGG

This is ideal for vegan baking. These "eggs" can replace real eggs in most recipes. I usually use 2:1 ratio of chia to chicken egg when replacing in a recipe. So, if a recipe calls for 1 egg, I'll substitute 2 flax "eggs" instead.

Makes 2 Eggs

---

2 tablespoons chia seeds or flaxseed

½ cup water

Mix seeds and water in a bowl and let sit for 25 minutes until they become jelly-like.

Use two flax eggs to replace each egg in a recipe.

ROOT ROAST

This is one of my go-to dishes, I always make it for the holidays, but it can be made any time of the year. You can play with the roots you use—I love adding in kabocha squash or delicata squash for different textures.

Makes 4 Servings

---

2 yams, washed and diced

2 beets, peeled, washed, and diced

5 carrots or parsnips, washed and diced

3 tablespoons coconut oil, melted

¾ teaspoon pink salt

Preheat oven to 400°F., and line a baking sheet with parchment paper.

Place all diced veggies in a large metal bowl.

Pour melted coconut oil all over vegetables and massage in the salt in with your hands.

Toss the vegetables on to the baking sheet and bake for 40 minutes or until tender and golden brown.

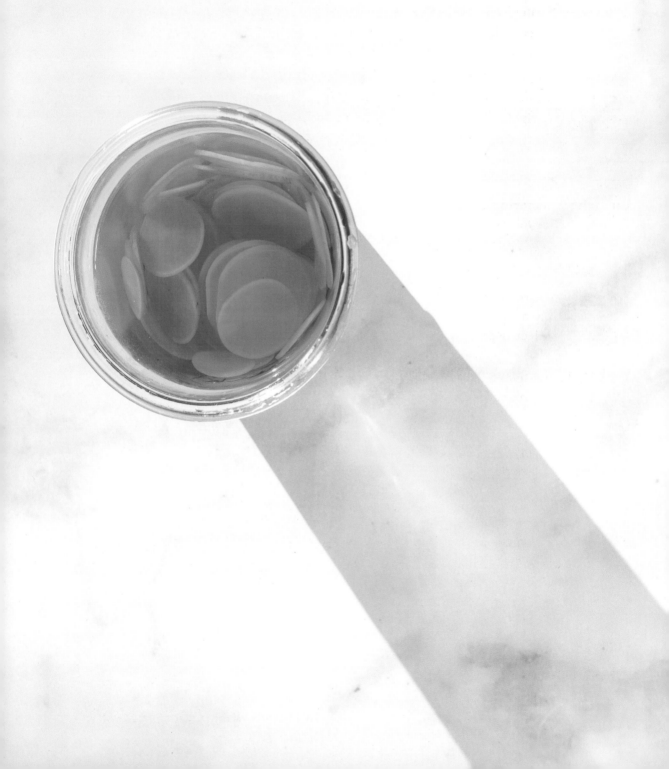

QUICK PICKLES

Quick pickles can give you a real kick of color and flavor in what could otherwise be considered a boring meal. I love them with beans, on my sweet potatoes, in salads, on sandwiches, or just out of the jar. Easy to make and delicious! They last a long time, so it's nice to make them in bulk. I play around with lots of different vegetables, but onions and radishes are my favorite. The turmeric and black pepper in the recipe makes them a powerhouse health food as well, helping to fight inflammation and build your immune system. I also opt for healthy apple cider vinegar instead of normal white vinegar. These are likely the healthiest pickles around!
Makes 4 Cups

---

for onion turmeric pickles

4 cups white or yellow onions,
   thinly sliced
8 cups water
1 cup honey
2 tablespoons turmeric powder
1 teaspoon cumin
1 tablespoon black pepper

for radish pickles

4 cups radish, thinly sliced
8 cups water
1 cup honey
1 teaspoon cumin
1 tablespoon black pepper

For whichever pickle option you're making, add all ingredients except your onions or radish to a large pot. Bring the water to a boil.

Add in your onions or radish and boil on high for 10 minutes.

Take off the stove and pour into 32-ounce canning jars.

Put the lid on and let cool.

Enjoy!

Keep refrigerated (will keep for months)!

NOTE: You can change out the turmeric powder for beet powder! This recipe also works great with cucumbers.

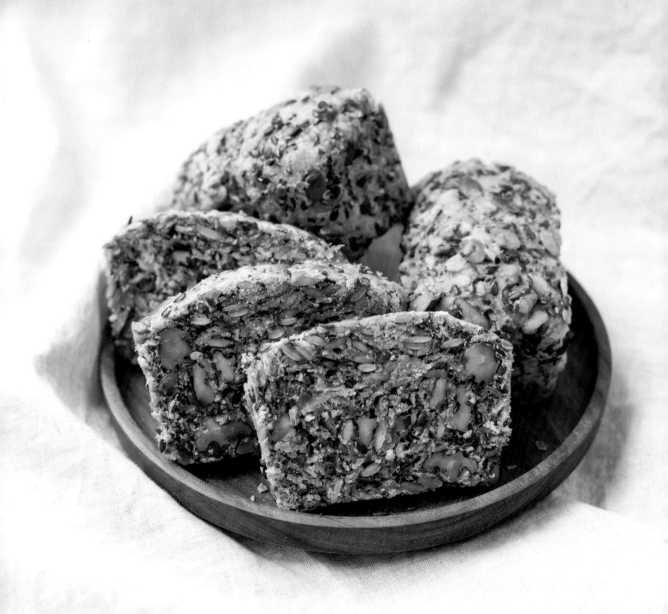

SIMPLE SEED BREAD

This bread is genius—we sell a version of it at Local Juicery. It's the perfect conventional bread alternative. The psyllium husk gives it a wonderful texture that is simply irresistible to me. These are some fun way to dress it up but honestly, fresh out of the oven with a nice slice of butter or coconut oil is divine.

Makes 5 Servings

½ cup flaxseed
½ cup hazelnuts
½ cup sunflower seeds
1½ cup sprouted oats
4 tablespoons psyllium husk
1 teaspoon salt
3 tablespoons coconut oil
3 tablespoons maple syrup
1¼ cups water

Preheat oven to 350°F.

In metal bowl, combine all dry ingredients, stirring well.

In a small bowl, whisk together maple syrup, oil, and water.

Add the wet mix to the dry ingredients and mix very well until everything is completely soaked and dough becomes very thick. Pour into your loaf pan.

Place pan in the oven on the middle rack, and bake for 20 minutes. Remove bread from loaf pan, place it upside down directly on the rack, and bake for another 10 to 15 minutes.

Keeps well for up to 7 days when refrigerated.

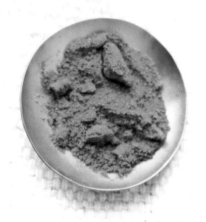

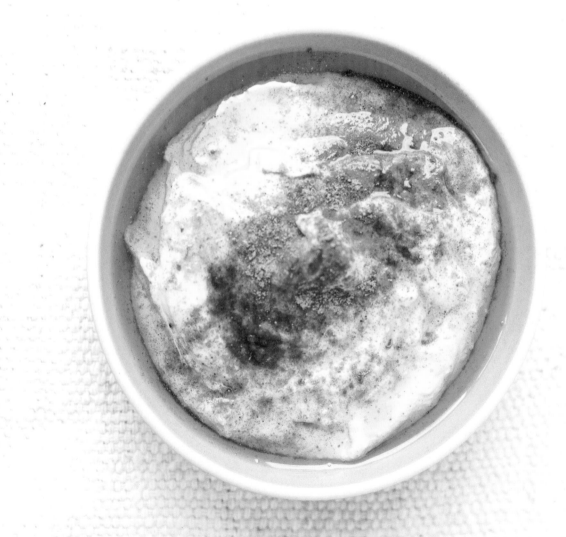

RAFFI'S HUMMUS

This recipe is inspired by a dear friend, Raffi. He's Syrian, and his food is amazing. I believe anything he touches turns to gold, and a lot of that is all the love he puts into whatever he does. This is a very creamy, very thick, very tahini-filled hummus inspired by him! It's always a hit. If you're planning ahead, it's nice to soak and cook your own garbanzos. I also buy them jarred from our local health food store.

Makes 8 Servings

3 cups cooked chickpeas
2 cups tahini
2–3 lemons, juiced
½ cup olive oil
1 teaspoon cumin
2–3 teaspoons salt
Cumin and paprika for topping

Combine all the ingredients in a high-speed blender and blend until very creamy. You may have trouble with the blender because this is so thick. I stop and stir the mixture every few seconds to help it move. You can add a tiny bit of water if absolutely necessary.

Pour into a bowl and top with cumin and paprika. You can also add a drizzle of olive oil on top!

CASHEW CREMA

Similar to the cashew cheese but with a smoother and with a consistency more like whipped cream. I highly recommend investing in a Vitamix if you are as obsessed with this nondairy cream option as I am.

Makes 12 Servings

1 cup soaked cashews
½–¾ cup water
2 tablespoons lemon juice
¼ teaspoon pink salt

Combine all the ingredients in a blender and blend on high until perfectly creamy.

Pour into a squeeze bottle or something easy to access for recipes.

NOTE: If you have a cashew allergy, you can replace with macadamia nuts or even blanched almonds.

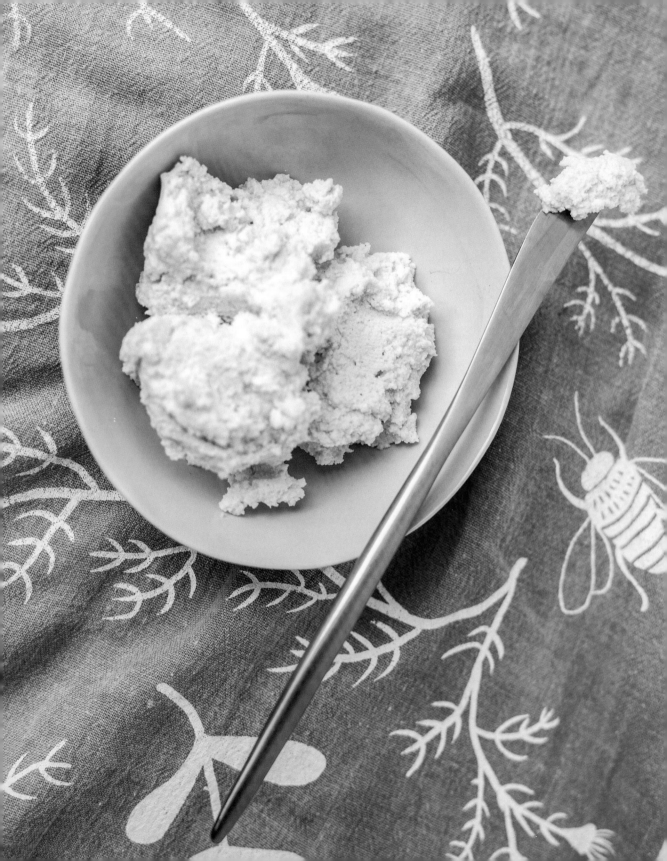

MACADAMIA NUT BUTTER

This is an absolute must-try. I adore this butter. It goes great on everything, especially nice baked yams!

Makes About 4 Cups

4 cups macadamia nuts
¾ teaspoon pink salt
½–¾ cup water
1 tablespoon coconut oil

Combine all the ingredients in a blender and blend on high until perfectly creamy. You may need to use a little extra water to get the blender going depending on the kind of blender you are using.

Keep in a glass container. This stores well for up to 1 week.

CASHEW CHEESE

This is a classic! It's a must-try in all kitchens, even if you eat dairy. A wonderful filling and side condiment to fancy up any meal. I love keeping this stocked in my fridge; I use it for almost every meal.

Makes 6 Servings

1 cup soaked cashews
½ teaspoon onion powder
½ cup nutritional yeast
½ teaspoon pink salt

Combine all the ingredients in a blender and blend on high until perfectly creamy. You may need to use a little water to get the blender going depending on the kind of blender you are using.

Note: If you have a cashew allergy, you can replace with macadamia nuts or even blanched almonds.

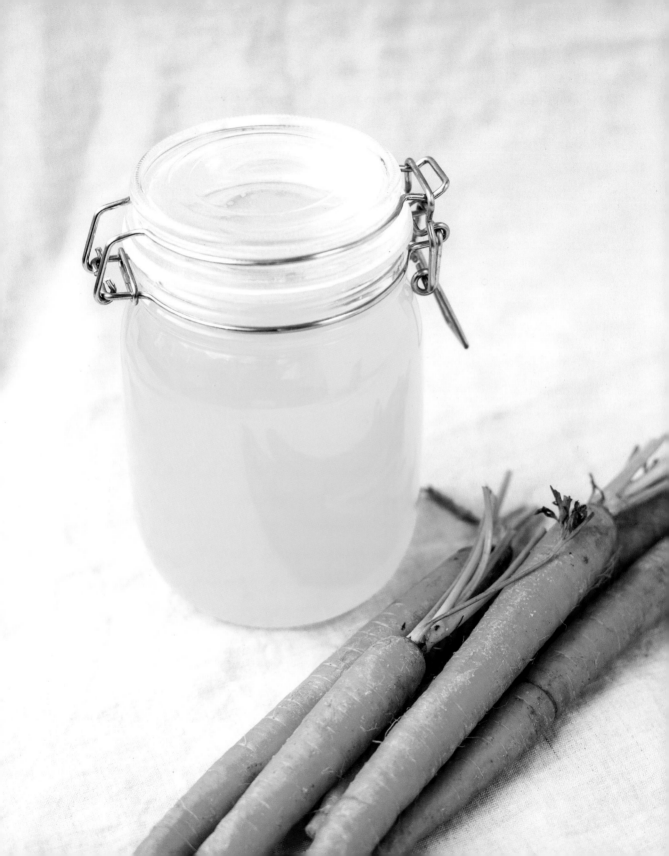

VEGGIE POTASSIUM BROTH

Potassium broth is great for increasing the mineral absorption in the body. It's a really nutritious option for before or after a workout or when you're healing from a cold.
Makes 8 Servings

6 potatoes, skin on, washed and
    diced
1 onion, chopped
4 carrots, chopped
6 celery stalks, diced
1 bunch parsley, minced
1 beet, with greens, chopped
1 clove garlic, minced
6 quarts filtered water

Place all prepared vegetables in a very large stockpot. Pour water in until covering vegetables.

Bring to a boil, then reduce heat and simmer for 45 minutes.

Remove from the heat and let the broth cool all the way.

Strain out the vegetables and store broth in a large mason jar. Broth will keep for about a week in the refrigerator.

CLASSIC PESTO

In my last book, *Raw and Radiant*, I focused a lot on patés and fun dips. You can find a couple different versions of pesto in it. This is a great way to easily fancy up any meal! It's simple and clean and pretty much everyone loves it. I like to use it on toasts or on stuffed sweet potatoes!
Makes 1½ Cups

¾ cup pine nuts
1 clove garlic, minced
3 cups basil, packed tightly
½ cup extra-virgin olive oil
1 teaspoon pink salt

In a food processor, combine the nuts and garlic. Pulse until ground.

Add in basil, olive oil, and salt. Pulse until well combined.

I like to keep mine a little chunky and less processed, but it is delicious either way.

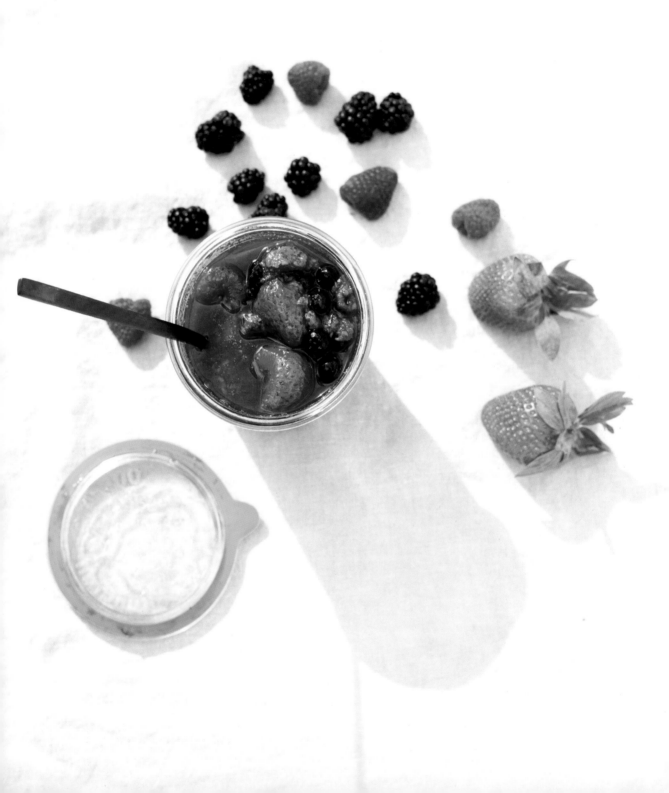

CLASSIC BERRY COMPOTE

A simple and delicious compote that can be made with a variety of berries for topping pancakes, French toast, or just eating out of the jar because it's so delicious!
Makes 8 Servings

---

3 cups strawberries, fresh or frozen
1 cup raspberries, fresh or frozen
¾ cup blueberries, fresh or frozen
½ cup fresh orange juice
1 tablespoon raw honey
Pinch of pink salt

Put all berries in a medium saucepan, and add in orange juice, honey, and salt.

Bring to a boil, stirring frequently, then turn to low and simmer for 5 to 10 minutes.

Let cool and then enjoy! Can be kept for up to 2 weeks in the refrigerator.

"RICOTTA"

A great replacement for regular ricotta or soft cheese. I love this in lasagnas, on taco night, or just as an add-on to salads or soups.
Makes 12 Servings

---

2 cups cashews, soaked
2 tablespoons olive oil
3 tablespoons nutritional yeast
½ teaspoon pink salt

Combine all the ingredients in a blender or food processor and blend on high until well blended and a ricotta texture forms.

Store in a glass container. This keeps for about 1 week.

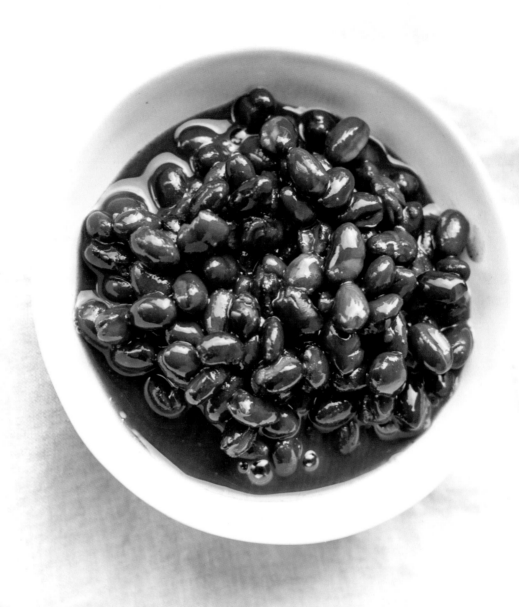

EASY BLACK BEANS

I have an old ceramic slow cooker from the 1970s. I refuse to buy a new one. I adore the ugly thing. My husband's parents received it as a wedding gift! I especially adore the black beans that come out of it. This is a recipe I make at least once a week. It's easy and can be used in so many ways. Try them in the Lettuce Wrap Tacos on page 220 or even added to pancakes for extra fiber!

Makes 6 Servings

3 cups soaked blacked beans
6½ cups water
2 tablespoons coconut oil
¼ cup maple syrup or honey
1 teaspoon chipotle powder
  (optional)
1 tablespoon pink salt

In a slow cooker or large cooking pot, add all the ingredients. Cook overnight for about 12 hours.

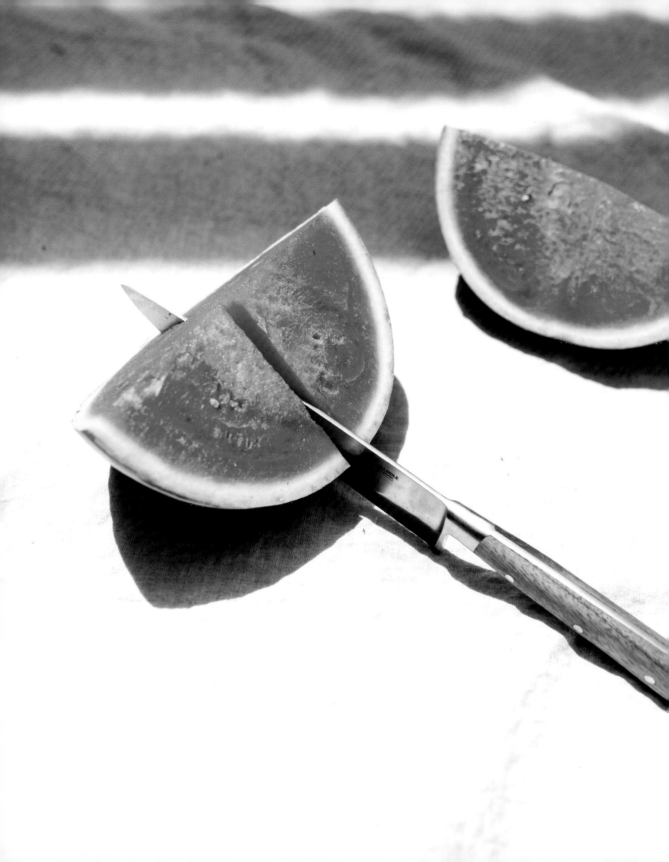

ON CLEANSING

TIPS FOR CLEANSING

A seasonal cleanse can be an incredibly beneficial ritual to incorporate into your life. Each season calls forth different energies from the earth and from within us. I find that a seasonal cleanse is not just a physical detox but also an emotional and spiritual reset. In the following pages, I've given you four different cleanses, each based on the season. As always, consult your physician before embarking on any diet change or cleanse.

STAY WARM

When we cleanse, especially with raw foods and juices, our bodies need more warmth. I like to take hot baths, sauna, steam, and stay cozy in blankets.

STOP CAFFEINE

It can be tempting to continue using caffeine while cleansing, because the detox side effects can be so challenging. If you want the full benefits of the cleanse, start weaning off coffee and heavy teas or any kind of soda at least a week before the cleanse. If you must have caffeine, opt for a clean version like an organic green tea.

ENEMAS

I go in depth on the importance of enemas and colon cleansing in my last book, *Raw and Radiant*, so I'll be keep it brief here. When you cleanse, especially with liquids, you don't have the fiber from the food moving things out, and it's incredibly important for toxins and old stuck feces to find their way out of your body. If you don't do colonics or at-home enemas, you run the risk of nasty breakouts and really terrible detox symptoms. Doing an enema will help everything move on out quickly. I suggest doing an enema or colonic every day to every other day during your cleanse.

DON'T BE HARSH

What I've found is when we get too strict and don't listen to our body's needs, we don't usually make it through a cleanse. The best thing to do is listen and feel. If you feel like you're starving, have an apple and some nuts, don't deny yourself what you feel you need so long as it's really a need and not just a craving.

BODYWORK

This is the time to love up on your body. If you can, schedule a lymph drainage massage or two. You can dry brush, do baking soda baths, and overall just pamper yourself. Take a peek at some ritual ideas on page 46.

IMPORTANT NOTE FOR ALL CLEANSES

Doing enemas or colonics daily is highly recommend, as is skin brushing. This will support your body in eliminating toxins. If you don't do this, you may see some breakouts or rashes. When your body doesn't have help eliminating, it will find a way!

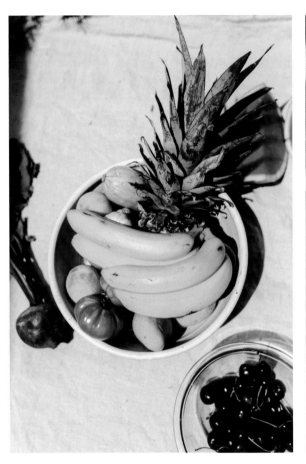
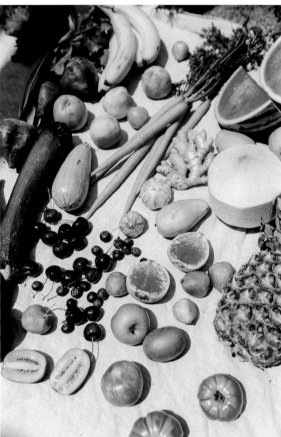

SPRING

March 21st to June 20th

Indulge | oranges, limes, grapefruit, lemons, kiwis, asparagus, spring greens, cauliflower, broccoli, sea veggies, quinoa

Limit | heavy foods such as meats, processed dairy, caffeine, and sugar

Spring Green Cleanse—6 days

This is a cleanse that includes some foods, but very light ones. This a full-body cleanse that will leave you looking amazing and feeling even better. The nutrients in this cleanse are otherworldly. Expect to glow. It is one of the more challenging cleanses because it is so *green*, but that's what makes it work. Nothing great comes easy.

What you'll need

6 lemons (1 per day)

6 oranges (1 per day)

6 grapefruits (1 per day)

5–6 pounds fresh sprouts (like alfalfa or sunflower)

Access to fresh wheatgrass or a powdered wheatgrass supplement

6 (16 ounce) organic raw (ideally cold-pressed) green juices **a day**. Think cucumber, celery, basil, spinach, kale, and a tiny bit of green apple if needed

A good mineral supplement for your water

A skin brush

Enema bucket or scheduled colonic

How to Cleanse

morning Each morning upon rising, drink a big glass of fresh water.

Juice 1 lemon, 1 orange, and 1 grapefruit together, and enjoy! This might take a bit of getting used to—it will be tart. That is the point. This will alkalize your body.

midmorning 1 cup sprouts with a bit of lemon and pink salt. Once you enjoy this, have your first green juice or two!

afternoon Now is a good time to take a bath or walk if your schedule allows. Drink another 1 to 2 green juices. This is also the time for your wheatgrass shot! If you're doing a dry powder, mix with 4 ounces of water and enjoy (if you can!).

evening Enjoy your last 2 green juices. If you find that you're needing to fill your stomach a little more, an apple or fresh fruit would be okay to add in to this part of your day.

SUMMER

June 21st to September 22nd

Indulge | berries, mango, melons, apricot, bitter greens, spinach, chard, peas, sprouts, fresh goat cheese
Limit | heavy foods such as meats, processed dairy, caffeine, and sugar

The Watermelon Fast—4–6 days

This is an incredible flush for your kidneys, gallbladder, and your overall body pH. You'll alkalize and flush out so much! I love this cleanse because watermelon is my most favorite thing in the world and because each time I do it I feel absolutely amazing. You'll balance out the acid in your body and bring back balance your kidneys. Don't forget to eat the seeds! Watermelon seeds naturally contain glutathione, which helps support and protect your body from oxidative stress. You may start drinking organic raw cold-pressed green juice on day 3 if you feel you need more.

What You'll Need

A large watermelon for each day you'll be fasting
A good mineral supplement for your water (I use Quinton from Quicksilver Scientific)
A skin brush
Enema bucket or scheduled colonic

How to Cleanse

This is a really simple cleanse—you really just feast on the melon when you feel hungry! I like to start the day with a big cup of fresh water with added minerals. Eat whenever you're hungry and drink when thirsty.

AUTUMN

September 24th to December 20th

Indulge | apple, pear, persimmon, dates, grapes, figs, pomegranate, brussels sprouts, ginger, collards, yams, sweet potatoes, oats, barley, thyme, beans, yogurt, pastured eggs

Limit | heavy foods such as meats, processed dairy, caffeine, and sugar

The Colon Cleanse—3–4 days

This is a fairly intense colon cleanse that is inspired by Dr. Bernard Jensen and his work with cleansing the bowels. Each day you'll make 5 to 6 shakes with the following ingredients.

What you'll need

½ cup apple juice

½ cup water

1 heaping tablespoon psyllium husk or powder

3 tablespoons bentonite clay liquid

A good mineral supplement for your water

A skin brush

Enema bucket or scheduled colonic

Raw cold-pressed green and fruit juice

How to Cleanse

In a jar with a lid, combine all ingredients. Shake rapidly for 15 seconds and then drink all of it. Follow with a cup of water if you can. Do this 5 to 6 times a day. You may notice when you do an enema that fecal matter will begin to come out that is dark brown, even black! It can look like ropes. Very bizarre but awesome because you know you're really cleansing.

Drink cold-pressed organic juices whenever you may feel hungry. You may also eat fresh sprouts, just be sure to clean them properly.

When your 4th day is complete, you can begin to add in some simple steamed vegetables or vegetable broth. Break your cleanse slowly—it's always recommended to be gentle with breaking a fast. Your body is in a pristine but delicate state. Treat it well.

WINTER

The Soup Cleanse—5 days

This is a heartier cleanse using warming soups and teas. The point is to get lots of vegetables and broth into your body. Soups are very easy to digest and the warmth is great for your organs.

What You'll Need

Favorite vegetables for soup (see recipes on page 189) or choose some of your own favorites, keeping it vegetable-based

Premade vegetable broth (making it yourself is always best), see page 263

A good mineral supplement for your water

A skin brush

Enema bucket or scheduled colonic

How to Cleanse

This cleanse is based on your personal favorite simple soup recipes. Keep it clean and simple! There are lots of soup ideas in this book beginning on page 189.

morning Each morning upon rising, drink a big 12-ounce glass of fresh water.

Start your day with miso soup with scallions or a gentle vegetable broth.

midmorning as much herbal tea as you would like.

lunch a simple soup of onion, garlic, broccoli, carrot, potato, yams, and spinach. Season with herbs of your choice, quality salt, and pepper.

evening enjoy a hearty soup made of steamed yams and blended with vegetable or bone broth, coconut milk, cinnamon, and pink salt.

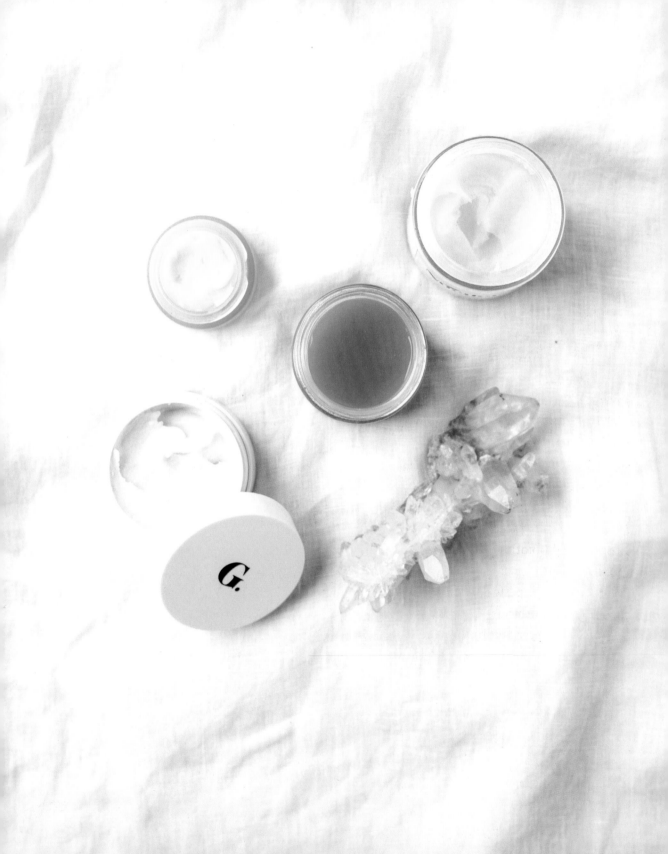

SOME FAVORITES

HEALTH + BEAUTY

2 Rise Naturals CBD

Anima Mundi Apothecary

Bee's Keeper Naturals Honey

Cap Beauty Products and Superfoods

Dr. Haushkha Rose Day Cream

Epic Protein Powders

Goop Beauty Skincare

HealthForce Superfoods

Heritage Store Rosewater Body Spray

Ilia Cosmetics

Inner-sense Beauty Haircare

Jiva Apoha Body Oils

Juice Beauty Skincare

Kosås Cosmetics

Living Libations Skincare

Moon Juice Superfoods + Adaptogens

Nucifera Balm Skincare

Sakara Life Probiotics + Nootropic
   Chocolates

Shaman Shack Superfoods + Adaptogens

Sun Potion Superfoods + Adaptogens

Vintners Daughter Serum Skincare

SKIN CARE + BODY SPECIALISTS

Tess Adams | Aesthetician NY + LA

Alice Dell | Alphabiotics Sedona

Adam Di Viro | Acupuncture Sedona

Lori Krass | Network Chiropractic Sedona

HEALERS + MOTIVATORS

KC Baker Woman's Speaking Coach

Carista Liminare Psychotherapist +
   Relationship Miracle Worker

Ashley Neese Breathwork Coach

Lacy Phillips Manifestation Coach

Katrine Volynsky Functional Health
   Specialist

Josephine Willieks Physic

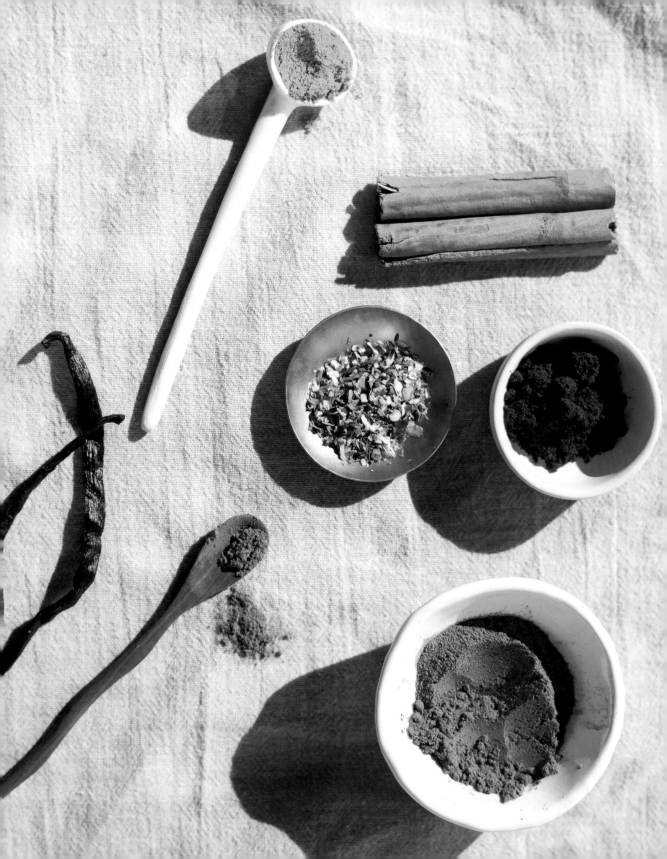

FAVORITE BOOKS

Anything You Want by Derek Sivers

Conscious Loving by Gay Hendricks, PhD and Kathlyn Hendricks, PhD

Do What Feels Good by Hannah Bronfman

Eat Clean, Play Dirty by Danielle Duboise and Whitney Tingle

Family Secrets by John Bradshaw

Goddesses by Joseph Campbell

Healing the Shame that Binds You by John Bradshaw

High Vibrational Beauty by Cindy DiPrima Morisse and Kerrilynn Pamer

Isis Mary Sophia by Rudolf Steiner

Money: A Love Story by Kate Northrup

Recovery by Russell Brand

The Body Keeps The Score By Bessel Van Der Klok

The Hormone Cure and Younger by Sara Gottfried

The Presence Process by Michael Brown

The State of Affairs by Esther Perel

The White Hot Truth by Danielle Laporte

Vaccines, Autoimmunity and the Changing Nature of Childhood Illness by Thomas Cowen, MD

Why We Sleep by Matthew Walker, PhD

Wired For Love by Stan Tatkin, PsyD, MFT

Woman by Natalie Angrier

WomanCode by Alissa Vitti

Women Who Run With Wolves by Clarissa Pinkola Estés

CONVERSION CHARTS

METRIC AND IMPERIAL CONVERSIONS

(These conversions are rounded for convenience)

Ingredient	Cups/Tablespoons/ Teaspoons	Ounces	Grams/Milliliters
Butter	1 cup/ 16 tablespoons/ 2 sticks	8 ounces	230 grams
Cheese, shredded	1 cup	4 ounces	110 grams
Cream cheese	1 tablespoon	0.5 ounce	14.5 grams
Cornstarch	1 tablespoon	0.3 ounce	8 grams
Flour, all-purpose	1 cup/1 tablespoon	4.5 ounces/0.3 ounce	125 grams/8 grams
Flour, whole wheat	1 cup	4 ounces	120 grams
Fruit, dried	1 cup	4 ounces	120 grams
Fruits or veggies, chopped	1 cup	5 to 7 ounces	145 to 200 grams
Fruits or veggies, pureed	1 cup	8.5 ounces	245 grams
Honey, maple syrup, or corn syrup	1 tablespoon	0.75 ounce	20 grams
Liquids: cream, milk, water, or juice	1 cup	8 fluid ounces	240 milliliters
Oats	1 cup	5.5 ounces	150 grams
Salt	1 teaspoon	0.2 ounce	6 grams
Spices: cinnamon, cloves, ginger, or nutmeg (ground)	1 teaspoon	0.2 ounce	5 milliliters
Sugar, brown, firmly packed	1 cup	7 ounces	200 grams
Sugar, white	1 cup/1 tablespoon	7 ounces/0.5 ounce	200 grams/12.5 grams
Vanilla extract	1 teaspoon	0.2 ounce	4 grams

OVEN TEMPERATURES

Fahrenheit	Celsius	Gas Mark
225°	110°	¼
250°	120°	½
275°	140°	1
300°	150°	2
325°	160°	3
350°	180°	4
375°	190°	5
400°	200°	6
425°	220°	7
450°	230°	8

SOAKING CHARTS

NUTS	
TYPE	**TIME**
Almonds	12 hours
Brazil	No need to soak
Cashews	2 hours
Filberts	No need to soak
Macadamia	No need to soak
Pecan	6 hours
Walnuts	4 hours

GRAINS	
TYPE	**TIME**
Buckwheat	2 hours
Corn	12 hours
Millet	8 hours
Oats	6 hours
Quinoa	5 hours
Rice	8 hours

SEEDS	
TYPE	**TIME**
Flax	8 hours
Hemp	No need to soak
Pepitas	8 hours
Sesame	8 hours
Sunflower	8 hours

LEGUMES	
TYPE	**TIME**
Adzuki	8 hours
Black beans	12 hours
Chickpeas	12 hours
Lentils	8 hours
Mung beans	12 hours

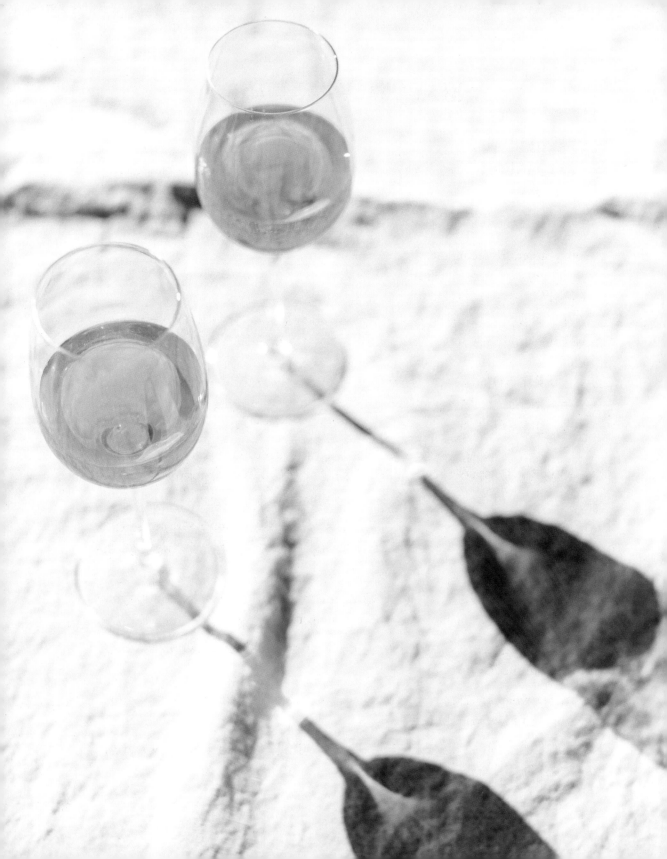

ACKNOWLEDGMENTS

MY FAMILY

My husband Mike for being okay with me buying crazy amounts of ceramics to make this book pretty! And for so much more than I can fit into this small area. I love you.

My son Henry, because nothing I've done would be tangible if not for you.

My mother, for teaching me.

My god father, for seeing me.

MY EDITOR

Leah, thank you so much for making my books actually books! You're such a love and I adore working with you. I can't wait for the next project.

DEAR FRIENDS + MENTORS

My dear friends for being there for me and always supporting in ways that have inspired aspects of this book.

Nate Hansen, I love you dearly my friend. I'm so happy to have you in my life. You edited my first book when it was just a dream. Thank you for supporting me in this life.

Lyrica Tyree, you are really, truly, to the core an artist. I respect you and your values so much. You inspire me to step back and look more at the full picture, but also to hone in on the details that are often missed.

John Mack, you've inspired me to think differently. I have so much respect for your heart and your mind. Thank you for always showing up fully.

Carista Luminare, for everything you've done for our family and your ability to see the needle in the haystack.

Alexa Gray, what a pleasure it is to know you and work with you. You are so talented and dear, and I love you dearly.

Kristin Dahl, your eye for real beauty and your depth of heart. I love you and am always inspired by your care for the world.

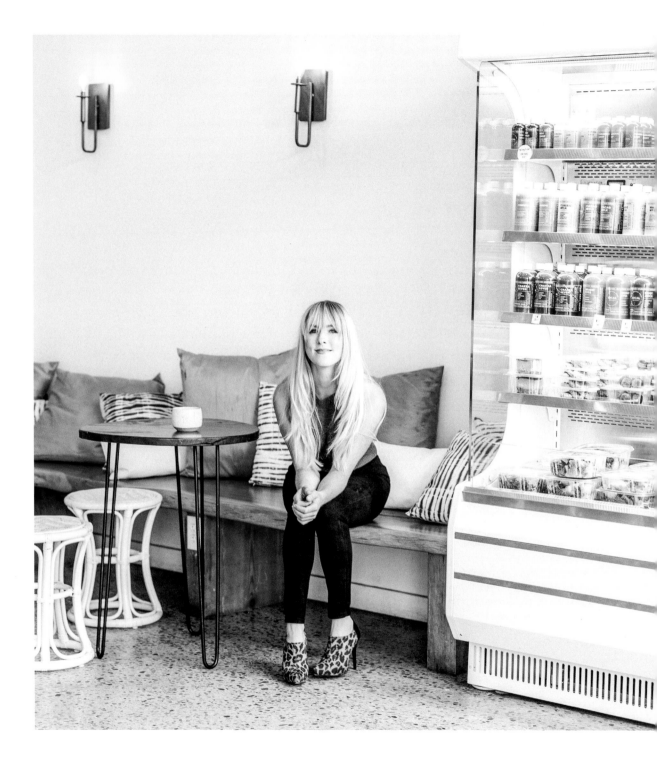

ABOUT SUMMER

Summer Sanders is a mother of two, plant-inspired chef, and founder of Local Juicery in Arizona. She is passionate about supporting women to live healthy, connected, and full lives. Summer is a trained raw food chef and worked closely with renowned raw food chef and restaurateur Matthew Kenney. She is a detox specialist, cosmetologist, certified personal trainer, and an overall natural living nerd. Summer lives in Sedona, Arizona, with her family, where she spends her time playing in the kitchen and developing new recipes for Local Juicery and enjoying the red rocks. She is the author of *Raw and Radiant*, and shares frequently with the online health community. Find more about Summer at www.strongandradiant.com

INDEX